THE
YOGA-BODY
CLEANSE

THE
YOGA-BODY
CLEANSE

A 7-DAY AYURVEDIC DETOX
TO REJUVENATE YOUR BODY
AND CALM YOUR MIND

ROBIN WESTEN

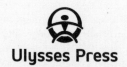

Ulysses Press

Published in the U.S. by
ULYSSES PRESS
P.O. Box 3440
Berkeley, CA 94703
www.ulyssespress.com

ISBN: 978-1-61243-279-3
Library of Congress Control Number 2013947594

Acquisitions Editor: Katherine Furman
Managing Editor: Claire Chun
Editor: Lauren Harrison
Proofreader: Elyce Berrigan-Dunlop
Front cover design: Rebecca Lown
Interior design and layout: what!design @ whatweb.com
Cover photograph: © ifong/shutterstock.com

10 9 8 7 6 5 4 3 2 1

Printed in the United States by United Graphics Inc.

Distributed by Publishers Group West

NOTE TO READERS
This book has been written and published strictly for informational and
educational purposes only. It is not intended to serve as medical advice or to
be any form of medical treatment. You should always consult your physician
before altering or changing any aspect of your medical treatment and/or
undertaking a diet regimen, including the guidelines as described in this book.
Do not stop or change any prescription medications without the guidance
and advice of your physician. Any use of the information in this book is made
on the reader's good judgment after consulting with his or her physician and
is the reader's sole responsibility. This book is not intended to diagnose or treat
any medical condition and is not a substitute for a physician.

With gratitude to Tara Glazier—
extraordinary yoga teacher, visionary founder, and owner
of Brooklyn's Abaya Yoga—who helped deepen my practice,
open my heart, and turn me on to the transformational
power of detox cleansing.

CONTENTS

INTRODUCTION

As a yoga practitioner and meditator for over 15 years, I've
noodled around with lots of esoteric and practical disciplines
while trying to get a hold of what this life, *my* life, is all about.
I figure, *here I am — GO FOR IT!*

I'm not alone in doing this. If you're reading *The Yoga-Body
Cleanse* right now, you've probably also explored the nooks
and crannies of your own being and in the process rooted
around in the forest of different schools of thought as to
how to approach your body. My explorations have taken
me to several Zen and Tibetan Buddhist monasteries on the
East Coast, a Balinese shaking energy adept, a hardcore tai
chi master in Manhattan, several healers around the country
including one who poked the top of my head with explosive
vigor, dozens of channelers (while writing a book on the
phenomenon). I've enjoyed time with a renowned Chinese
qigong teacher, accomplished acupuncturists and Reiki
practitioners, as well as lymphatic drainage, Swedish, Shiatsu,
hot stone, deep tissue, and Thai massage therapists. I've also
checked out brief stints of psychotherapy, chanted with yoga's
"rock star" Krishna Das, been hugged by the Indian saint
Amma, sat with Insight Meditation founder Sharon Saltzberg,

and joined a mind-blowing retreat in Maui with Baba Ram Dass, the author of my personal bible, *Be Here Now*. Or to put it another way, I've been around. And this is where I've landed.

My focus for the past several years has been on heart-opening yoga, introduced to me by Tara Glazier, the founder and owner of Abhaya Yoga, a light-splattered studio overlooking New York City's skyline and the powerful currents of the East River. I had been practicing yoga for at least a decade before then. But in those days, it was a physical pursuit with occasional insights. Mostly I practiced bringing my competitive nature to the mat. At Abhaya there was a total turnaround. It didn't happen overnight (if only change was so easy!), but slowly it dawned on me that opening, rather than forcing or even trying, was key. In the process, and over a couple of years, I experienced a new level of readiness—a growing and brilliant *emptiness*. I guess the old adage "Nature abhors a vacuum" is true, because I opened and became receptive, and in rushed expansive wonder.

Along with yoga, which resulted in periods of intense joy, I began to crave a more serious meditation practice. With not much fanfare, I found myself waking earlier and setting a morning schedule that includes, *without fail*, 30 minutes of sitting. My ritual involves simply lighting a stick of incense, placing a cushion on the floor in front of a small alter that displays a portrait of revered Hindu saint, Neem Karoli Baba, who continues to inspire my "trip," then settling down to breathe and watch my mind jump around. Sometimes my brain takes a break and when it does, again, there's a release, and again, an opening.

Simultaneously with this shift came a heightened awareness of my body's sluggishness. I noticed my energy was lagging, my emotional reactions too often teetering on a high wire, my digestive system slacking off; my skin was dull and my outlook flickered with negativity, anxiety, and fear. I suspected the cloudiness had something to do with my diet, so I cut back on sugary treats, coffee, gave up the morning croissant, and passed on a second glass of red wine with my evening meal. Yes, I noticed a difference. But these changes were hardly enough to turn my world around. But as "luck" would have it, an Ayurvedic (the traditional system of Indian medicine that treats and integrates the body, mind, and spirit using a comprehensive holistic approach) detox juice cleanse was announced at my yoga studio. I was the first to sign up and inwardly, I made a commitment to not only devote myself wholly to the cleanse, but to consciously add treatments to the program that would enable me to bring my life into sharper focus.

What you'll find within the pages of *The Yoga-Body Cleanse* is the culmination of my numerous experiences. Stuff that didn't work well in terms of diet, such as yogurt shakes or pampering treatments like dips in a hot tub, were nixed from the program. Others that rocked my world are emphasized, namely a foundational focus on Ayurvedic guidelines, restorative yoga poses, deep breathing, meditation, homemade natural pampering treatments, and most importantly, maintaining an introspective yet positive attitude. There are plenty of simple recipes to help move along the benefits of the cleanse as well as simple instructions for each of the daily practices. And because I'm someone who appreciates the energy offered by a cheerleading section, there's lots of encouragement, including upbeat affirmations and quotes from inspirational figures. When a boost is needed, tacking up a few thought-provoking words might help you stick to the cleanse, even move to the next level.

There are several quizzes included in the book. None of them are too taxing, but they reveal important aspects of your being and can help you figure out where you need to place special attention. For example, at the start of the *The Yoga-Body Cleanse* there's a quiz to identify which toxins are most prevalent in your daily life. As in the other tests that follow, there's an analysis that offers solutions to your personal issues. There's also a quiz to help you identify your Dosha, or nature, based on the three principles of Ayurveda: Vata, Pitta, and Kapha. This step will guide you to a deeper understanding of which treatments, foods, juices, meditations, and poses will be most effective for your cleanse. Whenever you take a quiz, it's a good idea to allow yourself time to approach the questions with serious consideration. Also, be honest with your answers. There are no right or wrong responses, only illuminating ones.

Before beginning the actual cleanse, you'll be offered tips on how to plan for your week ahead. There's a comprehensive shopping list with the foods and equipment needed for your menus and at-home pampering and relaxing sessions. Don't worry, none of it is very expensive or hard to find. At the end of the chapter you can get a picture of just how prepared you are by taking the "Are You Ready?" quiz. Should you need a few more days to prepare fully, it will serve you well to take them before rushing ahead. You'll know when the time is right.

Don't be surprised if lots of stuff shakes out during the course of the cleanse. Not only does your body release toxins, but your mind and emotions may be on a gallop. For this reason, besides the changes in your diet, a daily "activities" schedule is suggested; it will not only help to keep stress to a minimum, but also enhance your psychic and spiritual strength. For the first couple of days, you may rankle at the day's formality, but trust me, once you're in the flow you'll recognize how essential the regimen is to support the ease of your cleanse. Think of it as a mini retreat. Although you'll still be able to go to work, take care of your family, and fulfill other responsibilities with focus and commitment, you'll have the time to rise with the sun, start your day remembering your dreams, enjoy a 30-minute meditation, engage in a restorative yoga pose, and revel in the tastes and textures of the foods and juices you've chosen to consume.

After the seven days, I guarantee you'll feel a major shift: thoughts will be clearer and more creative, your digestive process will be speedier, your skin and hair will be glowing, your emotions will be on a steadier keel, and between 5 and 8 pounds (or more!) of weight will be dropped. Don't be surprised when folks who know you well remark on how fabulous you look.

But a few months down the road, you might feel like you need a pick-me-up. What if you don't have the time to commit to a seven-day event? Try out the Weekend Warrior Cleanse in Chapter Six. This 24-hour fasting approach promises a noticeable bump in how you look and feel. In the winter, I follow it one weekend a month. During warmer seasons I might do it two or even three times a month. The primary function of the shortened fast is to allow your organs to rest and go through a general, quick-fix housekeeping. You won't be "scrubbed clean" the way you are after a seven-day detox, but you'll definitely feel a difference. Even though you're fasting for only 24 hours, your stomach and intestines will shrink a bit. The excretion of digestive juices will decrease, and your intestines will change from being organs of absorption to organs of excretion. The excretion of waste products and toxins will also take place in the liver and other organs participating in the digestive system.

Ultimately, the goal is not only to look and feel better, but to embrace life with a renewed enthusiasm, to be positive in your moment-to-moment experiences, to approach change with curiosity, to open your heart without judgment to all beings including yourself, to tap into your personal source of energy, and to relax into the beauty of the world around you.

This may seem like a tall order—and it is. But as I learned, you'll never know what's really possible without wiping the dust from your lens. *The 7 Day Yoga-Body Cleanse* is a chance to do it. Go for it!

CHAPTER ONE

WHY CLEAN UP YOUR ACT?

"What we are doing to the forests of the world is but a mirror reflection of what we are doing to ourselves and to one another."

—Mahatma Gandhi

Because it's a dirty, messy, unhealthy world. Every day our bodies are bombarded with toxic elements: from food additives and preservatives, polluted water and air, dubious pharmaceuticals, poisonous cleaning and building products, and health-damaging cosmetics to hormone-infused meats and poultry, and mercury-laced fish—just to name the obvious culprits. Factor in our own toxic tendencies, which might include choosing an unhealthy diet, getting angry, feeling stressed, or blowing off exercise, and the wellness equation gets snarkier. Even though our liver, colon, kidneys, lymph system, and skin are designed to cleanse our bodies, the modern world and our unhealthy habits put way too much demand on them; it's impossible for our systems to keep pace. That's why it's sad but not surprising that:

- 🌱 one in every three adults is obese

- 🌱 8.3 percent of our population has diabetes

- 🌱 one in every ten Americans takes an antidepressant

- 🌱 one out of five Americans has an anger management problem

- 🌱 31 percent of our population has high blood pressure

- 🌱 up to 70 million U.S. adults have sleep or wakefulness disorder

- 🌱 50 million of us are suffering from allergies—FYI, that's more than any time *ever*.

Good for you if you if you read through this disturbing list and can honestly say you don't fit into *any* of these stats. But don't be lulled into thinking you're a hale, hearty, satiny rose in full bloom. If you drive or ride in a car, own a couch, feel stressed out, walk in the grass or dig around in a garden, order coffee at a café, shampoo your hair or brush your teeth with commercial products, get manicures and pedicures, drink beer or cocktails regularly, breathe our planet's air … okay, let's put it this way: If you are *alive*, don't be fooled. Poisons have accumulated in your body. Which means, among other reactions, your metabolism isn't functioning optimally; your skin is probably lackluster, you may be feeling edgy or fatigued, and sleeping through the night or enjoying a juicy sex life is most likely a shadowy memory.

On the following pages I'll describe common toxins to which we are most frequently exposed during our daily lives. Although this can seem like a hopeless downer, perhaps overwhelming, take heart. The amount of time toxins stay in our bodies is directly related to the balance between the amount of exposure and the amount of cleansing. In other words, you have a way out. Once you begin your cleansing journey, the reversal process will be set in motion. In the meantime, here's what you may be up against:

Surprising Enemies in Your House

CANDLES: Yes, burning them is romantic, but it's also filling you with toxins. To enhance candles' slow-burning effect, most (mainly those that are scented) have metal wires that contain lead inside their wicks. Lead has been associated with learning disabilities and Parkinson's disease. The artificial fragrances may also contain plasticizers and other solvent-type mixtures.

OVEN CLEANERS: It's not surprising there's a label warning us that the ingredients can burn our skin. Oven cleaners contain lye (also known as "caustic soda") ethers, ethylene glycol, methylene chloride, and petroleum distillates. Even spraying the aerosol contents involves releasing the neurotoxin solvent butane.

CARPETS: They contain dozens of harmful chemicals, including flame retardants, antistain ingredients, and volatile organic compounds. And that new carpet smell? Well, it's a carcinogen called p-dichlorobenzene, derived from 4-Phenylcyclohexene, and linked to visual, nasal, and respiratory problems.

DRYER SHEETS: Don't let commercials convince you that you need this product to have fresh-smelling laundry. Their synthetic fragrances include benzyl acetate, benzyl alcohol, and terpines—all are toxic and some are carcinogenic. Clothes tossed in the dryer along with these sheets absorb the harmful chemicals, and then we slip them against our skin. Not good.

TOXIC FURNITURE: Sure that couch or table was a bargain, but inexpensive particle-board, often called pressed wood, is typically made with formaldehyde or isocyanate glues. Both these glues are toxic, and the chemicals are released as gas and then inhaled. And brominated and chlorinated flame retardants, which are often found in upholstered furniture made with polyurethane foam, have been linked to cancer, neurological impairment, and hormone disruption.

Dangerous Fruits and Veggies

APPLES: Unless they're organic, an apple a day will not keep the doctor away. More than 40 different pesticides have been detected on apples because fungus and insect threats prompt farmers to spray various chemicals on their orchards.

BLUEBERRIES: These wonderful berries contain life-saving antioxidants, but they also have more than 50 pesticides. Your best alternative is to go organic.

CELERY: USDA tests have found more than 60 different pesticides on celery.

GRAPES: No matter whether they're green or purple, imported grapes can have more than 30 pesticides. Raisins also score high on pesticide residue tests.

LETTUCE: Along with spinach in the leafy greens category, lettuce makes the list of fruits and veggies with the most pesticides. More than 50 pesticides have been identified on lettuce.

PEACHES: More than 60 pesticides have been found on most peaches sold in supermarkets. A better option may be canned peaches, but the chemicals leaching from the can should give you pause.

POTATOES: Even though this is America's favorite vegetable, it still ranks high in pesticides. According to the United States Department of Agriculture (USDA), the common potato contains 35 pesticides. Opt for sweet potatoes, which have lower levels of residue.

SPINACH: This favorite of Popeye's is an excellent nutritional option if it's organic. If not, the leafy green will be grown with nearly 50 different pesticides.

STRAWBERRIES: To avoid fungus, farmers spray pesticides and their residue remains on berries sold at market. Almost 60 different pesticides have been found on strawberries. FYI: fewer are found on frozen strawberries.

Bad News Foods

FATTY RED MEAT: Pesticides linger in meat fat, and many of the dangerous chemicals are long-lived so they end up accumulating in our fat. The same pattern holds for other meats, with pork fat and chicken thighs tallying the most pesticide residue. Good news? Lean meat comes up innocent.

MILK: Pesticides and other man-made chemicals have been identified in human breast milk, so it should come as no surprise that they have been found in dairy products, too. Twelve different pesticides have been identified in milk.

COFFEE: Many of the coffee beans we buy are grown in countries with lax regulation. Look for the USDA label to ensure you're not buying beans that have been grown or processed with the use of potentially harmful chemicals.

WINE: Just like coffee (one of our favorite drinks!), there's no watchdog reporting on pesticides in wine, but grapes are among the crops that are typically heavily doused with chemicals to ward off fungus and bugs.

CHOCOLATE: Hate to be a killjoy, but cocoa beans are grown across the developing world, sometimes in countries without strict laws governing use of pesticides.

CANNED FOODS: Even if what's inside is organic, canned foods are dangerous. That's because they contain bisphenol A, a plastic and resin ingredient, which lines the metal food and drink cans. When the Centers for Disease and Prevention (CDC) did an analysis of BPA exposure they detected it in 92.6 percent of the people sampled, and noted that any Americans are exposed to bisphenol A at levels above the current safety threshold set by the EPA.

Processed Foods

WHITE FLOUR, RICE, PASTA, AND BREAD: If a whole grain is refined, it means most of its nutrients are destroyed in order to extend its shelf life. In the process, the bran and germ are removed as well as all the fiber, vitamins, and minerals. Because these stripped-down and refined grains are devoid of fiber and other nutrients, they can send your blood sugar and insulin skyrocketing, which can lead to all sorts of health problems.

HIGH-FRUCTOSE CORN SYRUP (HFCS): The amount of refined sugar we consume has declined over the past 40 years, but on the flip side, we're consuming almost 20 times as much HFCS. According to researchers at Tufts University, we take in more calories from HFCS than from any other source. That's terrible news because it increases heart-stopping triglycerides, boosts fat-storing hormones, and drives people to overeat and gain weight.

PALM OIL: Just like corn oil, when palm oil is blasted with hydrogen and turned into a solid, it becomes a trans fat. This process helps packaged foods stay "fresh." Eating junk food with trans fat raises your "bad" LDL cholesterol and triglycerides and lowers your "good" HDL cholesterol, ultimately increasing your risk of blood clots and heart attack.

SHORTENING: If you find a food that lists shortening or partially hydrogenated oil as an ingredient, don't eat it because it's also a trans fat. In addition to clogging your arteries and causing obesity, it also increases your risk of metabolic syndrome.

ARTIFICIAL SWEETENERS: Aspartame, saccharin, and sucrose may be even harder on our metabolic systems than real sugar. What's more, studies suggest that artificial sweeteners can trick our brains into forgetting that sweetness means extra calories, making us more likely to keep eating sweet treats.

SODIUM BENZOATE AND POTASSIUM BENZOATE: These preservatives are sometimes added to soda to prevent mold from growing, but benzene is a known carcinogen that is also linked with serious thyroid damage. Dangerous levels of benzene can build up when plastic bottles of soda are exposed to heat (left in the sun) or when the preservatives are combined with ascorbic acid (vitamin C).

BUTYLATED HYDROXYANISOLE (BHA): This chemical is a preservative that helps prevent spoilage and food poisoning. But it's also an endocrine disruptor that adversely affects your hormone balance.

SODIUM NITRATES: You'll find this preservative in processed meats like bacon, lunchmeat, and hot dogs. They're believed to cause colon cancer and metabolic syndrome, which can lead to diabetes.

ARTIFICIAL COLORING: Avoid blue, green, red, and yellow. They've all been linked to thyroid, adrenal, bladder, kidney, and brain cancers.

MSG: Monosodium glutamate is a processed "flavor enhancer." While glutamates are present in some natural foods, such as meat and cheese, the ones used by the processed foods industry are separated from their host proteins through hydrolysis. High levels of free glutamates have been shown to seriously affect brain chemistry.

Toxic Toiletries

TOOTHPASTE: The antibacterial and toxic ingredient triclosan is found in dozens of toothpaste brands. Triclosan is like a chlorinated pesticide, which means that it causes allergies and imbalances the immune system, just like other chlorinated pesticides.

NAIL POLISH: There are three terrible chemicals in conventional nail polish—toluene, dibutyl phthalate (DBP), and formaldehyde. Exposure to large amounts of these chemicals has been linked to developmental problems, asthma, and other illnesses

FRAGRANCE: Most perfumes are made with synthetic chemicals that are commonly synthesized from petroleum distillates. A study by the Environmental Protection Agency (EPA) found that numerous potentially hazardous chemicals are also commonly used in perfumes: acetone, benzaldehyde, benzyl acetate, benzyl alcohol, camphor, ethanol, ethyl acetate, limonene, linalool, and methylene chloride. When inhaled these chemicals can cause central nervous system disorders such as dizziness; nausea; slurred speech; drowsiness; irritation to the mouth, throat, eyes, skin, and lungs; kidney damage;

headache; respiratory failure; ataxia; and fatigue, among other reactions. In fact, the FDA reports that fragrances are responsible for 30 percent of all allergic reactions.

LIPSTICK: A recent study by the FDA found that 400 lipsticks contain lead. Plus, they contain other toxic chemicals that are responsible for nerve toxicity, endocrine disruption, and organ system toxicity.

Destructive Emotional Reactions

STRESS: Recent studies maintain that 75 to 90 percent of patients' visits to physicians are for ailments that have some kind of link with stress or anxiety. Stress begins in the brain with perceptions and emotions about a particular external event and ends up in the body as aches and pains, fatigue, headaches, heart palpitations, high blood pressure, hives, psoriasis, weight gain (or loss), and a host of other less common but more serious illnesses.

ANGER: According to Dr. Redford Williams, author of the landmark book *Anger Kills*, here's what happens to your body when you're angry: Aggressive thoughts percolate in your cerebral cortex sending out a wake-up call to a group of hypothalamic nerve cells deeper within the brain, where they cause outgoing nerves to signal the adrenal glands sitting on top of the kidneys to pump large doses of both adrenaline and cortisol into your bloodstream. As the adrenaline reaches your heart, it begins to pound faster and your blood pressure rises. What you don't feel is that the adrenaline is silently stimulating your cells to empty their contents into your blood stream and that your liver is converting fat into cholesterol. The result? High blood pressure, heart disease, and increased incidence of heart attack and stroke.

INSECURITY, ENVY, AND JEALOUSY: If we are insecure even when we have abundance, we are in effect investing our energy in the fear of future want. Our habit of comparing what we have now with what others possess produces this sense of insecurity, which denies us the capacity to enjoy what we have already and feel a sense of gratitude. Recent studies in the positive effects of gratitude have shown that it not only makes us happier but increases longevity. Dr. Robert Emmons, author of *The Psychology of Gratitude*, reports, "People who write down the things they are grateful for every day have stronger immune systems, more happiness, and less reaction to negative events."

DEPRESSION: Keep in mind that what we eat directly affects not only our physical health but our mental and emotional health also. When we are lacking in the right quantities of vitamins and minerals from fresh, unprocessed foods, or we're unable to absorb essential vitamins and minerals due to a poorly functioning body, we become more susceptible to conditions such as depression. And it has real consequences. Researchers at Duke University tracked heart disease and mood symptoms in 730 men and women over age 27 and found that people with symptoms of depression, such as hopelessness and low self-esteem, were 70 percent more likely to have heart attacks than those whose outlooks were cheerier.

At This Point, You Have a Choice

You can accept these conditions and your inevitable decline and continue existing without really experiencing the fullness of your life, or you can stop the wheels, reverse the process, and thrill once more to living. One of the best and quickest ways to get there is with *The Yoga-Body Cleanse*. Although it takes commitment, resolve, preparation, and follow-through, in only a week's time, you can drain your body of toxic forces and look forward to improved energy, clearer skin, shinier hair, improved digestion, better sleep, increased concentration, and a soul that soars with positivity. Did I mention you'll probably lose several pounds along the way?

But first, let's figure out the situation and find just where you stand on your personal toxicity scale. Even if your dietary, emotional, and environmental factors rate low in toxicity, the Yoga–Body Cleanse will revitalize your system and rid your body of harmful bacteria, viruses, and parasites, as well as bump up your energy. On the other hand, don't be discouraged if your score shows you're deep into a perilous zone. Use this knowledge as motivation to follow the Cleanse with utter devotion. No matter where the starting point, everyone will reach the same goal: bountiful rejuvenation, a clearer, more focused mind, and the ability to engage fully with the world around you. But first …

How Toxic Is Your Life?

To prepare for the following evaluation, I suggest you sit down in a quiet place, away from electronic interruptions and preferably in a natural setting—either outdoors or by a sunny window. Tell yourself that you deserve this uninterrupted time, and approach the task with wholehearted honesty.

Answer each question with Never, Occasionally, or Frequently.

DIET

1   When you're alone and boredom sets in, do you start to snack?
    O Never   Ø Occasionally   O Frequently

2   When planning meals, do you neglect to consider foods which foods you're serving that are low in unhealthy fats and additives?
    O Never   O Occasionally   O Frequently

3   Do you take into consideration whether produce is in season or grown locally?
    O Never   Ø Occasionally   O Frequently

4   If/when you eat Chinese food, do you do so without asking if it contains MSG?
    Ø Never   O Occasionally   O Frequently

5   When preparing a vegetable dish, do you feel so virtuous that you ignore what kind of fat you're cooking with?
    O Never   Ø Occasionally   O Frequently

6   When you experience a letdown, do you dig into that container of ice cream?
    Ø Never   O Occasionally   O Frequently

7   Do you frequent fast food restaurants?
    O Never   Ø Occasionally   O Frequently

8   Are you more likely to choose something gooey and rich rather than a bowl of fresh berries on a dessert menu?
    O Never   Ø Occasionally   O Frequently

9   Do you pass up the organic section of produce aisles to save money?
    O Never   O Occasionally   Ø Frequently

10 Do you quench your thirst with an ice-cold soda rather than water or cold-pressed juice?
    Ø Never   O Occasionally   O Frequently

11 Do you eat fruit without washing or peeling the skin?
    Ø Never   O Occasionally   O Frequently

12 Do you stop at the candy counter before going into a movie theater?
    O Never   O Occasionally   Ø Frequently

13 Do you drink more than one cup of coffee or caffeinated tea a day?
    O Never   O Occasionally   Ø Frequently

14 Do you buy foods without checking the labels or ingredients?
    O Never   Ø Occasionally   O Frequently

15 Do you drink more than one glass of alcohol regularly?
    Ø Never   O Occasionally   O Frequently

ENVIRONMENT

1 Do you use products designed to kill household pests like ants, roaches, and fleas?
   O Never   Ø Occasionally   O Frequently

2 Do you use lawn or garden products that are chemically based?
   Ø Never   O Occasionally   O Frequently

3 Do you have wall-to-wall carpeting?
   Ø Never   O Occasionally   O Frequently

4 Are you around a fireplace, wood stove, or kerosene heater?
   Ø Never   O Occasionally   O Frequently

5 Do you get manicures or pedicures?
   O Never   Ø Occasionally   O Frequently

6 Do you polish your furniture with commercial polishes or aerosol sprays?
   Ø Never   O Occasionally   O Frequently

7 Is your furniture covered with fabrics made from polyester, plastic, or other unnatural blends, and/or has it been treated with flame retardants?
   O Never   O Occasionally   Ø Frequently

8 Do you use commercial cleaners in your home that contain ammonia, bleach, artificial fragrances, or formaldehyde as their active ingredients (check the labels)?
   O Never   O Occasionally   Ø Frequently

9 Do you use conventionally produced shampoo and hair conditioner, deodorant, soap, toothpaste, and mouthwash rather than organic?
   O Never   O Occasionally   Ø Frequently

10 Do you sleep on no-iron bed linens?
   ○ Never   ○ Occasionally   ⊘ Frequently

11 How often do you get your clothing professionally cleaned?
   ⊘ Never   ○ Occasionally   ○ Frequently

12 Do you keep electronics like a computer, a cell phone, or an
   alarm clock right next to your bed?
   ○ Never   ○ Occasionally   ⊘ Frequently

13 Do you use indoor air fresheners or deodorizers?
   ⊘ Never   ○ Occasionally   ○ Frequently

14 Do you smoke indoors or allow others to do so?
   ⊘ Never   ○ Occasionally   ○ Frequently

15 Have you purchased (or rented) a house without checking for
   radon? (Not applicable for apartment dwellers.)
   ○ Never   ○ Occasionally   ⊘ Frequently

Take a Break

Before responding to the next group of questions, sit quietly
and do nothing but breathe deeply for five minutes. When
your mind is at peace, ask yourself, "Who am I?" Become
aware of the conflict between who you have been taught to
think you ought to be and who you really are.

Turn inward without judgment.

STRESS

1 Crowds make you feel a little edgy.
   O Never   O Occasionally   Ⓧ Frequently

2 You always have to be on time.
   O Never   O Occasionally   Ⓧ Frequently

3 You need to check things several times before you're satisfied.
   O Never   O Occasionally   Ⓧ Frequently

4 You worry about past mistakes.
   O Never   O Occasionally   Ⓧ Frequently

5 You find it hard to relax.
   O Never   O Occasionally   Ⓧ Frequently

6 You know it's unreasonable, but you still feel responsible for
   others' unhappiness.
   O Never   O Occasionally   Ⓧ Frequently

7 Planning for a trip causes you more anxiety than excitement.
   O Never   O Occasionally   Ⓧ Frequently

8 You don't feel like there's enough time in the day.
   O Never   O Occasionally   Ⓧ Frequently

9 You worry about your finances.
   O Never   O Occasionally   Ⓧ Frequently

10 You would describe your work as pressured.
   O Never   Ⓧ Occasionally   O Frequently

11 If you're fearful that you might create a problem, you don't say
   what you really mean.
   O Never   O Occasionally   Ⓧ Frequently

12 You don't have a lusty sex life.
   O Never   O Occasionally   O Frequently

13 You block out your feelings.
   O Never   O Occasionally   Ø Frequently

14 If your to-do list isn't completed at the end of the day, you feel like a failure.
   O Never   O Occasionally   Ø Frequently

15 You feel yourself getting agitated or tense without any good reason.
   O Never   O Occasionally   Ø Frequently

ANGER

1 When your feelings are hurt, you need at least a few hours (sometimes much longer) before you can talk about it.
   O Never   Ø Occasionally   O Frequently

2 How often do you feel disappointed or annoyed with your friends?
   O Never   O Occasionally   Ø Frequently

3 After a couple of drinks do you become silent, gloomy, or aggressive?
   Ø Never   O Occasionally   O Frequently

4 When you have a hard day, do you take your annoyance out on the people closest to you?
   O Never   Ø Occasionally   O Frequently

5 If a store clerk is rude to you, do you display rudeness in return?
   O Never   O Occasionally   Ø Frequently

6 When waiting for an elevator, do you press the button several times?
   O Never   Ø Occasionally   O Frequently

7 Do you experience road rage?
   O Never   O Occasionally   Ø Frequently

8 If you get in a heated argument, can you feel your heart pounding and breath becoming labored?
   O Never   O Occasionally   Ø Frequently

9 Do you find it hard to apologize?
   O Never   Ø Occasionally   O Frequently

10 Do you believe you're right most of the time?
   O Never   Ø Occasionally   O Frequently

11 Do you storm out of rooms to end an argument and have the last word?
   Ø Never   O Occasionally   O Frequently

12 Do you have high blood pressure?
   Ø Never   O Occasionally   O Frequently

13 Someone bumps into you on a crowded street; even though you know it's unintentional, do you still feel irritated?
   O Never   O Occasionally   Ø Frequently

14 When you're very angry at an individual, do you hit or shove him or her?
   Ø Never   O Occasionally   O Frequently

15 If someone criticizes you or treats you unfairly, are you likely to think about it for hours and imagine your revenge?
   O Never   O Occasionally   Ø Frequently

INSECURITY, JEALOUSY, AND ENVY

1 When your partner shows an interest in someone else, do you worry?
  O Never   O Occasionally   Ø Frequently

2 Do you believe that if the person who has fallen in love with you discovers the real you, it's all over?
  O Never   O Occasionally   Ø Frequently

3 You've gained 10 pounds. Will you refuse to go out socially until you've lost the extra weight?
  O Never   O Occasionally   Ø Frequently

4 If a friend recounted her vacation in great detail, would you respond by telling her all about the one you took?
  Ø Never   O Occasionally   O Frequently

5 Do you spend time gossiping?
  O Never   Ø Occasionally   O Frequently

6 When talking to new acquaintances, do you find yourself comparing their clothes, figures, and jewelry to your own?
  O Never   Ø Occasionally   O Frequently

7 If a colleague is promoted, are you likely to be unable to get over your resentment that you weren't?
  Ø Never   O Occasionally   O Frequently

8 Do you believe others don't appreciate your good qualities?
  O Never   O Occasionally   Ø Frequently

9 Do you believe celebrities have perfect lives?
  Ø Never   O Occasionally   O Frequently

10 Do you ever get the feeling that you're a "pretender"?
  O Never   O Occasionally   Ø Frequently

11 Do you spend more than an hour getting dressed before you're ready to go out for the day?
   Ⓧ Never   ◯ Occasionally   ◯ Frequently

12 Do you feel competitive with your friends?
   ◯ Never   Ⓧ Occasionally   ◯ Frequently

13 Do you ever wish you were living someone else's life?
   ◯ Never   ◯ Occasionally   Ⓧ Frequently

14 Do you tell lies or embellish the truth when talking about your childhood or present life?
   ◯ Never   ◯ Occasionally   Ⓧ Frequently

15 Do you check your partner's pockets, e-mail, social media, and/or credit card statements?
   Ⓧ Never   ◯ Occasionally   ◯ Frequently

DEPRESSION

1 You can't seem to concentrate long enough to finish tasks.
   ◯ Never   ◯ Occasionally   Ⓧ Frequently

2 Does your future feel hopeless?
   ◯ Never   ◯ Occasionally   Ⓧ Frequently

3 Have you ever been unable to finish a book.
   ◯ Never   ◯ Occasionally   Ⓧ Frequently

4 Is it tough for you to make a decision?
   ◯ Never   ◯ Occasionally   Ⓧ Frequently

5 Do you have a hard time falling asleep or staying asleep through the night?
   ◯ Never   ◯ Occasionally   Ⓧ Frequently

6   On that note, is it difficult for you to get out of bed in the morning?

O Never   Ø Occasionally   O Frequently

7   Are the activities that once interested you no longer appealing?

O Never   O Occasionally   Ø Frequently

8   Would you describe yourself as unhappy?

O Never   O Occasionally   Ø Frequently

9   Do you find yourself nervous for no reason at all?

O Never   O Occasionally   Ø Frequently

10 Do you feel exhausted?

O Never   O Occasionally   Ø Frequently

11 Do you have to use all your resources just to do something simple like shop for groceries or pay your bills?

O Never   O Occasionally   Ø Frequently

12 Do you feel like a failure?

O Never   O Occasionally   Ø Frequently

13 Is it especially difficult for you to socialize, especially around happy people?

O Never   O Occasionally   Ø Frequently

14 Have you recently gained or lost 10 pounds for no apparent reason?

Ø Never   O Occasionally   O Frequently

15 Do you ever have suicidal thoughts?

O Never   O Occasionally   Ø Frequently

Before Moving On

Congratulate yourself for completing the evaluation section.
Now total your scores from all the quizzes.

ANSWERS

	Never	Occasionally	Frequently
DIET	_____	_____	_____
ENVIRONMENT	_____	_____	_____
ANGER	_____	_____	_____
STRESS	_____	_____	_____
JEALOUSY, INSECURITY, AND ENVY	_____	_____	_____
TOTAL	_____	_____	_____

What Your Score Means

If your highest score is in the NEVER category, kudos!
Your level of toxicity is lower than most Americans. You
probably naturally gravitate toward a healthy diet and a clean
environment, and you've worked on your emotional reactions.
What's more, you've dealt with past traumas and for the most
part, let them go. Following the Yoga–Body Cleanse will be a
piece of cake. Oops! Hold that metaphor! Rather, it won't be
particularly challenging. Scan your results to focus on those

areas that are most toxic for you and keep them in mind during the Cleanse.

If you've landed mostly in the middle range, OCCASIONALLY, you're like most of us, aware that you should be taking steps toward a healthier lifestyle, but you may not have made the committed effort that this cleanse will offer you. Or, you might have tried other cleanses that haven't quite done their job. Here is your chance to take the reins and really improve your life. You might experience some unpleasantness at the start of the program as your body begins to adjust to the Yoga-Body Cleanse. These affects will disappear by the third day. Look over your test results again to see which areas in your life need special attention.

What if you've scored most often in the FREQUENTLY column? Well, the Yoga-Body Cleanse may be a challenge, but think of it this way: You'll benefit most from the amazing results. You're probably experiencing any number of issues from headaches, sleeplessness, and frequent colds to uncomfortable menstrual cycles, indecisiveness, and maybe even anxiety and depression. Let yourself imagine how much better you're going to feel! Trust me, it will be epic. Try not to skip any steps in the preparation section. Your body needs to get ready in earnest for its transformation.

CHAPTER TWO

ALL ABOUT AYURVEDICS

When diet is wrong, medicine is of no use.
When diet is correct, medicine is of no need.

— Ayurvedic Proverb

In the Beginning

"The Ayurvedics" sounds like a rock band, right? Well, in a sense this holistic health system that integrates our mind, body, and spirit has the same potential to put us in-sync with our body's natural rhythm. But unlike, let's say, The Ramones, it's been around long before electric guitars; in fact, long before *any* kind of electronics came on the scene. According to ancient Indian scripture known as the Vedas, the foundation of Ayurvedics was revealed as far back as 5,000 years ago by Lord Brahma, whom Hindus believe to be the creator of the universe. The word "Ayurveda" is derived from the combination of the words *Ayush* and *Veda*. Ayush means life, livingness, and liveliness, and Veda means perfect, complete knowledge.

Even though the original ancient Ayurvedic texts were either stolen or destroyed (thanks to relentless invasions of India), native doctors were able to preserve most of its knowledge and it's been passed down over the centuries, from generation to generation, as well as all over the word. In ancient times, the Chinese, Tibetans, Greeks, Romans, Egyptians, Afghanis, and Persians traveled to India to learn about Ayurvedic medicine and brought it back to use in their own countries. Later, Ayurvedics became popular in Europe and helped to form the philosophy of their present-day approach to medicine. That's because in sixteenth-century Europe, Paracelsus, who is known as the father of modem Western medicine there, practiced a system of healing which he borrowed mainly from Ayurveda. More recently, in the last few decades, there's been a revival of these ancient practices, especially in the United States.

According to Karta Purkh Singh Khalsa, author of *The Way of Ayurvedic Herbs*, Ayurveda is based in two medicinal and surgical instructions still in use today—the Charaka Samhita and the Sushruta Samhita. The Charaka Samhita is a compilation of internal medicine. It details the elemental principles of Ayurvedic therapeutics and is the only text to describe Ayurveda comprehensively. The Sushruta Samhita details surgical instruments and their use in Ayurvedic medicine. Anatomy, toxicology, and pharmacology are also described in the Sushruta. Over 650 natural remedies written centuries ago in the Sushruta Samhita are used by present day Ayurvedic practitioners.

Soul Sisters and Brothers

Ayurveda also contends that before we existed in a physical
form, we existed in a more subtle form known as the soul.
The ancient seers of India believed that we were composed of
a certain energetic essence that precluded our physical selves.
In fact, they believe that although we may occupy many
physical bodies throughout the course of time, our underlying
self, or soul, remains unchanged. This may explain why so
many people have experienced the sensation of being "out of
their bodies."

The Yoga Connection

Talk about a perfect match. When the Ayurvedic system
is experienced through a yogi's perspective, it generates
profound physical and emotional healing, inner bliss, and
clarity of mind, which in turn can overpower and cure
physical imbalances and mental neurosis. Together, Ayurveda
and Yoga offer ways to prevent and heal various disorders,

as well as to cleanse and rejuvenate the body. Both practices advocate the use of:

DIET: concentrating on the consumption of whole grains, fruits, nuts, and vegetables

HERBS: using a plant's seeds, berries, roots, leaves, bark, or flowers for medicinal purposes

ASANAS: practicing yoga postures

PRANAYAMA: consciously controlling the breath

MANTRA: repeating a sound, syllable, word, or group of words considered capable of creating transformation

PRAYER: invoking a rapport with a deity, an object of worship, or a spiritual entity through deliberate communication

PUJAS: making offerings like flowers, rice, incense to various deities, distinguished persons, or special guests

Some of these practices may seem too woo-woo and over-the-top for you, but keep in mind it's not necessary to do everything during your 7-Day Yoga-Body Cleanse. Following the diet, however, is crucial. Breath control, postures, herbs, and prayer won't hurt, either.

Ayurvedics and the Importance of Cleansing

Traditional Ayurvedic teachings recommend a program of dietary cleansing at each change of the seasons. The purpose is to clear out any buildup of toxins that occurred during the previous season. This allows the body to begin again, refreshed and renewed. Although ideally undertaken at the start of a season, the Yoga-Body Cleanse can be done any time of year. However, no matter what the season, it's important to always follow the Ayurvedic guidelines for reducing *ama*.

So What Is Ama?

According to *Eat-Taste-Heal: An Ayurvedic Guidebook and Cookbook for Modern Living*, "If water and blood are the sweet nectars of the body, ama is the rotten sludge." Ama is the undigested food residue that lodges itself within the organs and channels of our body. Ick!

Outward Signs of Ama:

- 🌿 White coating on your tongue when you wake in the morning

- 🌿 Fatigue

- 🌿 Poor appetite or cravings for junk food

- 🌿 General lack of motivation or zest for life

- 🌿 Feelings of heaviness or constipation

Ama Reducing Guidelines:

- 🌿 Do not fast or skip meals during any part of the 7-Day Yoga-Body Cleanse

- 🌿 Eat at the same time every day to keep your metabolism fired up

- 🌿 Eat while sitting down

- Sit quietly for a minute at the start of the meal. It's a good time to say a little prayer of gratitude or to breathe deeply.

- Pay attention to the food while you eat (no reading, watching television, or checking e-mails)

- Wait for a few minutes before leaving the table to give your digestion a chance to settle before your metabolism starts up

- If possible, eat with company and engage in pleasant conversation

- Don't eat until you're full. Stop at ¾ of your capacity

Doshas

Ayurvedic teachings profess that we all come into this world with our own unique energy design that is in charge of our mind, body, and emotional well-being. These energy designs are called "Doshas" and there are three types: Vata, Pitta, and Kapha. Identifying your Dosha, or your true nature, will help you to choose the foods, yoga postures, level of cleanse, and other practices, like meditation, massage, chanting, and breath control, that will benefit you most.

This quiz helps you identify your most predominant Dosha.

WHAT'S YOUR DOSHA?

1   I usually solve problems by:
    a. Thinking spontaneously outside the box
    b. Considering all angles before coming to a decision
    c. Letting someone else make a decision

2   My moods can be described as:
    a. Changeable
    b. Generally happy
    c. Prone to the blues

3   When it comes to learning new things, I'm:
    a. Quick to pick it up
    b. Would rather stick to my old ways
    c. Slow-paced

4   Sleeping straight through the night:
    a. Is just a dream—I wake throughout the night
    b. Is erratic—sometimes I'm like a hibernating bear, other times I have
       a hard time falling and staying asleep
    c. Mission always accomplished

5   My weight is:
    a. No problem. In fact, I have a tough time gaining weight (most of my
       friends are very annoyed!)
    b. Remains steady even though I have a healthy appetite
    c. A problem. I gain it way too easily and have a tough time dropping
       extra pounds.

6   My inner thermometer is:
    a. Chilly
    b. Hot
    c. Cool

7   My fingers are:
    a. Long
    b. Medium
    c. Shortish

8 I'd describe my complexion as:
   a. Dullish
   b. Rosy
   c. Pale

9 My hair is:
   a. Dry and brittle
   b. Thin
   c. Wavy and thick

10 Overall my body type is:
   a. Long, lean and lanky
   b. Medium with an athletic build
   c. Broad and more thick than thin

11 Under stressful circumstances, I'm more likely to be:
   a. Anxious or worried
   b. Irritable or aggressive
   c. Withdrawn or reclusive

12 My joints are:
   a. Thin and have a tendency to crack
   b. Loose and flex
   c. Large and well padded

13 My eyes appear:
   a. Smallish and always on the move
   b. Penetrating and focused
   c. Big and puppy doggish

NOTE: Mostly everyone possesses attributes of all three Doshas, but usually one is dominant. Your strongest Dosha will influence your entire being from your physical strengths and weaknesses to your personality's preferences and aversions. To get a picture of your dominant Dosha, total your scores and discover whether you're a Vata, Pitta, or Kapha.

If You Ccored Mostly A's, Your Dosha Is Vata

Creative, spontaneous, and full of fiery sparks, you can keep anyone engaged with your quick wit and facile mind. Plus, you're a brainiac, a superfast learner. On the flip side, you're so busy gaining new knowledge and diving into the latest fad that you sometimes forget the lessons you've learned—even those that should be kept. For example, you *know* you should eat less sugar and more protein, but you're more into getting a quick energy boost just to keep going. This means you often grab something sugary or a cup of coffee, then overexert yourself and subsequently feel totally wiped out. Most Vatas are slender, tall, and likely to walk at a fast clip (no surprise!). And you're usually bundled up even when it's not that cold outside because you don't have much meat on your bones and your hands can feel like ice cubes. Similarly, your hair and skin may be on the dry side and you're unlikely to break into a sweat. Vatas enjoy a good time and are quick to laugh, but your moods can quickly go from sunny to blue. You may also have a tendency to have high levels of anxiety, especially when your body is out of balance.

FAMOUS VATAS: Cameron Diaz and Nicole Kidman

QUICK TIPS FOR VATA

- Try to eat and sleep at the same time every night.

- Choose foods that are warm, cooked, nourishing, and easy to digest. Sweet berries, fruits, small beans, rice, and all nuts and dairy products are good choices.

- Exercise intensity should be moderate. A more meditative yoga, tai chi, walking, and swimming are all good options.

• •

If You Scored Mostly B's, Your Dosha Is Pitta

Focused, self-confident, and smart, you have all the attributes of a successful entrepreneur. That's because you love a challenge and are passionate about what you want. Put romantic interests in that mix. Physically, you're strong with a medium build and a hearty appetite. Your digestion is also top-notch and you rarely have to deal with tummy issues. What puts you on edge? Missing a meal. When you get stressed out, rather than experiencing nerves or breathless anxiety, you'll probably feel irritated and impatient. Most Pittas have fair skin, and that's why you may burn easily in the sun. Hey, why do you think you have freckles? Heat is also fatiguing and you perspire a lot. Typical physical problems include rashes or inflammations of the skin, acne, boils, skin cancer, insomnia, and dry or burning eyes.

FAMOUS PITTAS: Madonna and Julianne Moore

QUICK TIPS FOR PITTA

- Stay chill — avoid too much sun.

- Nix fried and spicy foods as well as alcohol. Instead, choose fresh vegetables and fruits that are watery and sweet, especially cherries, mangoes, cucumbers, water melon, and avocado. Have lots of salads with dark greens such as arugula, dandelions, and kale.

- You know about your quick-trigger temper, so try to avoid conflicts and practice honesty, generosity, and self-control.

• •

If You Scored Mostly C's, Your Dosha Is Kapha

Since you're so mellow and easygoing, mostly everyone loves to be around you. Stable, reliable, affectionate, and full of heart, your true nature is compassionate and forgiving. Plus, you have a ton of energy! And it doesn't just come in quick bursts. It's steady and strong. You may have a heavier build than other Doshas but your constitution allows you to approach every challenge with steadfastness. You speak slowly and deliberately wanting everyone to hear exactly what you mean. In return, you listen carefully and thoughtfully consider what's being said. It takes you a while to pick up new lessons, but once you learn they stick in your memory like Krazy Glue. Your appearance includes soft hair and creamy skin. Kaphas also tend to have large "puppy dog" eyes and sweet, soft voices. On the downside, your digestion can be sluggish and you're prone to depression. Other physical problems include colds and congestion, sinus headaches, and respiratory problems including asthma and allergies. But overall you're in excellent health with a superstrong immune system. The secret may be your gentle and breezy approach to life.

FAMOUS KAPHAS: Oprah Winfrey and Jennifer Lopez

● ●

QUICK TIPS FOR KAPHA

* To avoid sluggishness, weight gain, and the blues, make exercise a daily part of your routine.

* Be open to change and welcome in spontaneity!

* Eat foods that are light, warm, and spicy. Avoid heavy oily and processed sugars. Use lots of spices such as black pepper, ginger, cumin, chili, and lots of bitter dark greens.

● ●

The Five Elements

Ayurvedic medicine not only concentrates on the three Doshas but it also emphasizes the five elements, or major forces, responsible for keeping us healthy and in balance: ether, air, fire, water, and earth. These elements are listed in order from the subtle, light, and intangible, to the heavy, dense, and gross; each element acts in a specific way. In Sanskrit this system is known as the *Pancha Maha Bhuta* (*Pancha* means "five," *Maha* means "great," and *Bhuta* means "elements"). In essence, the five elements cover *everything* that makes up the universe. When in balance, these five essential elements sustain life. But when out of balance they not only create discomfort but can also, according to Ayurvedic medicine, threaten life. Here's a breakdown of each element:

1 ETHER: This is the place where all objects of the universe exist. Modernist physicists confirm that matter is a manifestation of ether and energy; contemporary Ayurvedic scholars believe ether is like nuclear energy and its unseen stored potential. Its qualities are clear, light, subtle, soft, and immeasurable.

2 AIR: The main principle of air is movement. Any time there is motion, we know air must be present. Within the body, it predominantly manifests as the electrical energy in the nervous system, movement of all tissues and cell functions, and the formation of gases. It governs all of the senses due to its affinity with the nervous system and specifically the sense of touch and the action of the hands to give, receive, and move things.

3 FIRE: This element represents transformation and metabolism. Within the body it predominantly manifests as the fire of intelligence and comprehension, balance of body temperature, the absorption and assimilation of food, and the transformative power of the liver. The blood carries the properties of fire through the body.

4 WATER: The main focus of water is transportation. Within the body it manifests as the plasma and lymph which transports nutrients to the cells and takes toxins away from them. Water governs the sense of taste and the action of reproduction through the genital organs.

5 EARTH: Anywhere there is stability, permanence, and rigidity there will be a dominance of earth. It cradles and holds all creatures of the planet, giving them support, food, and shelter. Within the body it predominantly manifests as the solid structures such as bones, muscles,

cartilage, nails, hair, teeth, and skin. Earth governs the sense of smell and the action of excreting waste products.

Become Sense-Able

When all the five human senses—taste, touch, sight, sound, and smell—are in harmony and properly nourished, you feel healthier. This is a common principle in Ayurveda and in the practice of yoga. Each of the senses in Ayurvedic philosophy is based on the notion that they can be stimulated to experience the world in a more vibrant way. Which sense is most tuned in depends on the individual. Some people enjoy listening to music, while others revel in the taste of food or watching a field of wildflowers sway in the breeze. Stepping into the world of sensual experiences is encouraged by both practices.

The Chakras

Both Ayurveda and yoga philosophy adhere to the existence of seven basic chakras, or energy centers located in the body. If any chakra is blocked and the energy isn't flowing freely, it negatively affects our physical health and our emotional and spiritual well-being. Traditionally, Ayurvedic practitioners see the body as arranged vertically from the base of the spine to the top of the head. *Chakra* is the Sanskrit word for "wheel," and these "wheels" are thought of as spinning vortexes of energy.

Each chakra is connected to particular life experiences. The openness of our individual chakras will determine how we approach and interpret these experiences. Chakras can be affected not only by external situations but also by our internal habits, including long-held physical tension and how we inwardly view ourselves. Not surprisingly, it's important to keep our chakras open, whirring, and balanced.

Sometimes chakra imbalances are temporary and can be the result of a passing situation like a relationship difficulty or a tough day at work. Other times, imbalances are chronic, and these usually develop from childhood issues, profound physical or emotional traumas, or intense and lingering pain. Regardless of the cause, with the Yoga-Body Cleanse coupled with specific yoga postures, meditation, mantra, and visualization practices, chakras can be restored to a healthy flow and balance.

FIRST: The Root Chakra is at the base of the spine (tailbone) and represents our foundation and sense of feeling grounded. It deals with issues of physical survival, safety, and security, and is blocked and weakened by fear and insecurity. The first chakra acts as a pump at the base of the chakra system that helps energy rise and flow. If this base pump is weak, work done on the other chakras won't be as effective.

SECOND: The Sacral Chakra is in the lower abdomen (approximately two inches below the navel) and represents our ability to accept others and new experiences. It allows us to "go with the flow" and open to pleasure and growth. It's also associated with the hips, sacrum, lower back, genitals, womb, bladder, and kidneys, and is connected with sexuality, emotions, and desire. Think orgasm and tears.

THIRD: The Solar Plexus Chakra is in the upper stomach area and represents our sense of confidence and ability to be in control of our lives. This chakra is involved in self-esteem, warrior energy, and the power of transformation. Plus, it governs digestion and metabolism. It's from this chakra that our deep belly laughter emanates, as well as authentic warmth and the yearning to perform selfless service.

FOURTH: The Heart Chakra is in the center of the chest just above the heart and represents our ability to love and connect with others and the universe. Through the heart chakra, we open to harmony and peace. Within our heart lives wholeness, boundless love, and a wellspring of compassion.

FIFTH: The Throat Chakra represents our ability to communicate. The fifth chakra resonates with our inner truth and helps us find a personal way to speak our truth to the outside world. The rhythm of music, creativity of dance, the vibration of singing, and the communication we make through writing and speaking are all fifth chakra ways to express ourselves.

SIXTH: The Third Eye Chakra is on the forehead between the eyes and represents our ability to see "the big picture" beyond the self. It awakens our ability to connect psychically to the world around us. While our two eyes see the material world, our sixth chakra sees beyond the physical. This vision includes clairvoyance, telepathy, intuition, dreaming, imagination, and visualization.

SEVENTH: The Crown Chakra is at the very top of the head and represents our ability to connect on a deep, spiritual level. It symbolizes the highest state of enlightenment and facilitates our spiritual development. The seventh chakra is like a halo atop the head.

But You're Not All That

Despite the Ayurvedic philosophy of unifying principles, the system also views each person as wholly individual with a unique mind–body constitution, personality, life circumstances, and emotional blueprints. You can think about it in the same way that scientists today consider DNA to be the foundation of the individual. We're all different, and yet there are unifying forces within all of us. And because we each have a unique constitution, our health prescription must be unique to us. This means that in order to be healthy, you need to eat certain foods that are beneficial for your body type and stay away from others. Your best exercise program should be personally suited as well. Your individual constitution also determines your personality and how you relate to other people. In this way, your emotional responses and personality are all yours.

Our lives are not in the lap of the gods, but in the lap of our cooks. — Lin Yutang

CHAPTER THREE

THE SEVEN SUPPORTS

"Fear less, hope more; Eat less, chew more; Whine less, breathe more; Talk less, say more; Love more, and all good things will be yours"

—Swedish proverb

Imagine the number seven is the whole enchilada, stuffed with powerful significance. Let's take a few bites and chew over its auspiciousness. For instance, the ancient Egyptians had *seven* original and higher gods; the Phoenicians *seven kabiris* (deities); the Persians, *seven* sacred horses of Mithra; the Parsees had *seven* angels opposed by *seven* demons, and *seven* celestial abodes paralleled by *seven* lower regions and their *seven* gods were often represented as one *seven-headed* deity.

The ancients believed that heaven was subjected to the *seven* planets; that's why in nearly all the religious systems we find *seven* heavens. The priests of many Oriental nations were subdivided into *seven* degrees; *seven* steps led to their altars and in their temples burnt candles in seven-branched candlesticks.

The Seven Supports   57

Several of the Masonic Lodges have, to this day, *seven* and *fourteen* steps. In the *Rámáyana* (one of the great epics of India that forms an important part of the Hindu literature), *seven* yards are mentioned in the residences of the Indian kings; and *seven* gates generally led to their famous temples and ancient cities.

The Christian Middle Ages studied *seven* free arts (grammar, rhetoric, dialectics, arithmetic, geometry, music, astronomy). In fact, during the Middle Ages, an oath had to be taken before *seven* witnesses, and the one to whom it was administered was sprinkled *seven* times with blood. The processions around the temples went *seven* times, and the devotees had to kneel *seven* times before uttering a vow. The Mahometan pilgrims turned around Kaaba *seven* times at their arrival, and their sacred vessels were made of gold and silver purified *seven* times.

Today's numerologists agree seven represents the seeker, the thinker, the searcher of truth who doesn't look at the world superficially and instead attempts to understand the underlying hidden truths. Those who are ruled by the number seven know that nothing is exactly as it seems and that reality is often hidden behind illusions. Although seven is spiritual (it's the energy of the mystics), in most numerologists' views it's not necessarily religious. In fact, the age-old questions of what life is all about, why we're here, and who we are, are essential to the seven's life-experience.

Beginning with the Seven Days of Genesis and following with the Seven Seals of Revelation, the Bible offers numerous references to the power of the number seven. According to this scripture, on the seventh day God ended his work and rested. But note: Though creation was ended on the Seventh

Day, it was just the beginning of the rest of the work for those on earth.

Hopefully, by now you realize it's no coincidence that your Yoga-Body Cleanse is carried out for seven days, and it also includes seven crucial steps. Each one leads to a deeper cleansing experience, so try them out in order. You may be surprised at the power of this seven-step preparation.

Step One: Intention

Everything begins with intention. When you hold an intention, it gives you the ability to bring your awareness to the bigger picture and secure it, not only in your mind, but also in your heart. In order to access the extraordinary power of intent, it's important to realize that it operates in a limitless field of energy; it's beyond—way beyond—a simple thought.

The initial step to supporting your higher consciousness so that you can revel in the benefits of cleansing is simply to have the intention to do it. Part of the process of setting an intention is to be aware how easily we can get caught up in the usual pressures of daily life: caring for loved ones, paying bills, working, housekeeping, etc. You can still accomplish your daily responsibilities while cleansing as long as you set your intention to open to your vast, endless energy.

In other words, if your intention is to follow the 7-Day Yoga-Body Cleanse and gain its rewards—you will.

Once your intention is embedded in your being, you'll feel its power. You can now trust that fulfillment of your desire is possible. Relax into the knowledge that the outcome you intend is right here, right now.

● ●

INTENTION BUILDERS

Ask yourself:

- How strong is my intention right now?
- What behavior or belief do I need to release so that my intention can be even stronger?
- When I focus on my intention, what part of my body is awakened?

● ●

Step Two: Affirmations

I'll try this cleanse, but knowing me, I probably won't be able to stick to it.

I wish I did, but really, I have no self-discipline.

I'm addicted to junk food.

Sound familiar? Most of us have a judgmental mind. Rather than urging us to succeed, it tells us we can't do something; we're just not good enough. We're too lazy, tired, anxious, stressed out, unhealthy, or scattered to accomplish our goal. This kind of negative thinking sabotages our self-confidence, our mood, and our commitment to change. And negative thinking can be self-fulfilling. That's why you want to banish these downer thoughts. End the loop! Shake up your brain waves!

How? By using positive affirmations: specific statements that help you to overcome self-sabotaging, negative thoughts. Affirmations will help you visualize and believe you can succeed with your 7-Day Yoga-Body Cleanse. These uplifting statements will support positive changes in your life. And it's not just a lot of New Age baloney; there are studies to support the power of positive affirmations.

For instance, a study by researchers at Northwestern State University in Louisiana found that people who used positive affirmations for two weeks experienced higher self-esteem than at the beginning of the study. Also, in a study published in the *Journal of American College Health*, researchers found that women treated with cognitive behavioral techniques that included use of positive affirmations experienced a decrease in depressive symptoms and negative thinking. A study by researchers at the University of Kentucky, Lexington, had similar results, and came to a similar conclusion.

So here's the deal. Try repeating three positive affirmations every single morning and every evening. Speak them out loud as you look at yourself in the mirror, record them in your own voice on your mobile phone and listen to them before you go to bed, or write them down on a piece of paper and put them on your bathroom mirror or refrigerator. Whatever works for you. The best affirmations are the ones you create for yourself. But if you're feeling a little brain blocked, here are some starters:

- 🌿 I'm happy with myself for following the 7-Day Yoga-Body Cleanse.

- 🌿 It makes me feel good to be completely free of pain and sickness and to be eating a well-balanced diet of natural foods.

- 🌿 I feel proud of my body and confident that I will feel great from this day onward.

- 🌿 I see myself as decisive and self-assured.

- 🌿 I will be thinner, healthier, and more energetic.

Step Three: Making Time for Yourself

"What day is it?"
"It's today," squeaked Piglet.
"My favorite day," said Pooh.

— A.A. Milne

These seven days are devoted to *you*. Even so, if you're like most of us, your day is so hectic that even with the best intentions you may not believe you'll be able to follow through on this week-long journey of purification. But you can do it by planning for your cleanse in advance.

Check off seven consecutive days on your calendar when you're unlikely to have an ultrastressed mental or physical schedule. It's ideal if you can set aside vacation time. If not, be certain that family, friends, and coworkers are aware of your endeavor. For added encouragement, consider this: According to a recent *Real Simple*–GFK Roper happiness study, 65 percent of women who say they're "very happy" make time for themselves. (Only 39 percent of women who are "somewhat happy" do so.) The odds are good that the more time you make for yourself, the happier you'll be. Here's how to do it:

Write down how you *really* spend your time: You might be shocked by how little time you spend doing things you love most. The key question to ask yourself is this: *"Am I spending my time on things that are good for my mind, body, and spirit?"*

SLOW DOWN: Reducing stress and hypermental activity is one of the key ways to be successful with your cleanse. If you're habitually rushing around and overscheduling, it's not only affecting your mind and your mood, but also your physical strength. Instead, meditate, breathe deeply, do your relaxing yoga poses, take warm baths or saunas, get a facial, book a massage, walk by the sea, or stroll down a country road.

• •

TIP

It's a good idea to wake an hour earlier than usual during the cleanse. You'll need this added time to meditate, prepare foods, do your yoga poses, and enjoy the sunshine.

• •

Reset Your Clock: Rise with the sun. Tuck in by ten.

DELEGATE: You'll need some help during this week, so why not ask your colleagues, partner, even your kids (if you have them) to help out? Think about it. If you can hand over a task, you've got that much more time to devote to yourself. If you've reflexively been doing most of the household duties, turn some of them over to your partner. Try similar strategies at work. Or make an investment and outsource. Just for this week, if housekeeping is important and there's no one to help out, hire someone or do a bartering deal.

ELIMINATE DISTRACTIONS: Shut the door. No kidding, if you have work to do, make it clear that you need to be left alone. At work, check your e-mail only twice a day. At home, give your cell phone a rest. As for TV, watch a show you love, and then turn off the set.

Practice paying attention to your present moment: "Ordinary thoughts course through our mind like a deafening waterfall," writes Jon Kabat-Zinn, the biomedical scientist who introduced meditation into mainstream medicine. In order to feel more in control of your mind and your life, to find the sense of balance that eludes most of us, you need to step out of this current, to pause, and, as Kabat-Zinn puts it, to "rest in stillness — to stop doing and focus on just being." In other words, we need to live more in the moment. Reminding yourself to quiet your mind and revel in the now will be especially helpful as you prepare for your week-long cleanse.

AND REMEMBER: *"Lost time is never found again."* — Benjamin Franklin

Step Four: The Shopping List

While you're cleansing you probably won't want to spend much time wandering around food stores, or any stores for that matter. So, do as much shopping in advance as possible. Here is a list offered by my yoga teacher, Tara Glazier, the owner of Abhaya Yoga in Brooklyn, New York. She suggested we gather these items before we embarked on our class cleanse, and I hope it will be just as helpful for your adventure as it was for me.

NOTE: Whenever possible, shop at an organic market and/or farmers' market that carries whole foods and supplements.

Recipe Ingredients:

1 Cold-pressed olive oil and/or cold-pressed flaxseed oil (in refrigerator section)

2 Dark leafy greens (kale, chard, dandelion, spinach, etc.)

3 Healthy grains (brown rice, jasmine rice, black rice, quinoa, millet, etc.)

4 Basmati rice (for kitchari)

5 Ghee

6 Mung beans (for kitchari)

7 Fresh, bright salad fixings (lettuce, cucumber, peppers, onion, etc.)

8 Raw nuts and seeds

9 Broccoli, carrots, zucchini, bell peppers, asparagus

10 Avocados

11 Lemons and/or limes

12 Fresh gingerroot

13 Turmeric powder

14 Mustard seeds

15 Whole cumin seeds

16 Celtic sea salt or Himalayan salt

17 Ginger tea

18 Fresh cilantro

19 Seaweed (for soup)

20 Ground cardamom

21 Ground cinnamon

22 Garlic

23 Olives

24 Gluten-free oats

Snacks (optional):

1 Organic flaxseed and brown rice crackers

2 Popcorn kernels

3 Seaweed snacks

4 Fruit: Pick fruits that are fresh and in season, but limit how many you get and never eat them for breakfast—they are only if you're dying for a sweet.

Supplements (optional):

1 Triphala (an Ayurvedic herb for health)

2 Organic, cold-pressed oil for Abhyanga

3 Probiotics

4 Fish oil (cod liver in liquid form) or algae capsules

5 Spirulina or E3Live: the only form of blue algae that is frozen and harvested at peak times. It has more chlorophyll than any other food. If you are feeling weak, uninspired, or addicted to coffee or stimulants, this is the supplement for you. It's available at most health food stores in the refrigerator section.

6 Aloe vera juice

Equipment:

1 Tongue scraper to remove ama (page 43)

2 Body brush to scrub dead skin

3 Journal or notebook to record thoughts, revelations, dreams

4 Unscented beeswax candles

• •

CONTEMPLATING A JUICER?

First things first: You don't need a juicer for the Yoga-Body Cleanse, and certainly not a fancy one. A sturdy blender will do. No problemo. But maybe you've been dreaming about getting a juicer, and who am I to mess around with that? Well, at least let me say my piece.

Only invest in a juicer if you're actually going to be using it. You're probably thinking "Duh. Of course I'm going to use it!" Trust me, it's how you're feeling now. From what I've heard, there are quite a number of juicers collecting dust in cupboards and on counters from coast to coast.

So, here's what I suggest. If you definitely want one, start off buying a cheap centrifugal juicer. This is the kind with blades that spin at a high speed and shave, then pulverize, your fruits and vegetables. After this step, the pulverized "mush" passes through a fine metal mesh screen that separates the fiber from the juice. You'll have to cut your fruit into itty bitty pieces and it may die on you after a year's heavy use. But I promise you'll consider it worth every penny. Now you can upgrade in confidence if you're still a juice fan.

FYI: The Good Housekeeping Research Institute tested 24 models of juicers and chose the Breville Juice Fountain Elite as the best all around one. Reviewers say it's fast and quiet, pointing out that it's made of strong stainless steel. It has two speeds and a wide feed tube, and all removable parts (except the food pusher) are dishwasher-safe. It minimizes mess by dispensing directly into a detachable pitcher. Cost? Around $300. But let me be clear, this is not my recommendation. I'm Switzerland when it comes to products. Neutral.

• •

Step Five: Setting Up Appointments

Remember in Step Four how I mentioned you probably won't be in the mood to go shopping while you're on the Cleanse? Well, you probably won't be in the frame of mind to be on the phone, or in front of your computer, setting up appointments either. That's why you'll want to arrange your life as much as is possible before the Cleanse begins so you have time to prepare your meals, luxuriate in relaxation, limit distractions, avoid hassles, move inward, and open to the shiny shift in your consciousness.

The following are several treatments I recommend you book in advance and enjoy during your week-long cleanse. They can be costly, so you might consider a barter system. Hey, if you have a partner who enjoys giving massages—lucky you. Go for it! But you may also want to book a special detoxing lymphatic-drainage massage. Read more about this type of massage below.

There are, however, two things to watch out for:

🌿 Only choose pampering that involves nontoxic, natural products. This probably means no salon manicures or pedicures. If you're going for a massage or facial, check with the practitioner before booking your appointment to be sure all their lotions are nontoxic.

🌿 When making appointments for treatments such as acupuncture, lymphatic drainage massage, and Reiki, be sure the practitioners are professionally licensed or certified.

Here are some of my favorite treatments to indulge in while detoxing:

SAUNA: If you belong to a gym that has a sauna, now is the time to make use of it. If not, most health facilities will let you use the one on their premises for a fee. It's worth it. In medieval times, healers relied on saunas to cure illnesses, and priests used their heat to chase away evil spirits. An old Finnish saying describes the sauna accurately as a "sacred place, a place of silence, a place of recreation, a place of peace, and a place of health." Why resist this powerful house of sweat?

● ● ● ● ● ● ● ● ● ● ● ● ● ● ● ● ● ● ●

SAUNA GUIDELINES

- Speak with your doctor if you have any health problems to determine if a sauna is safe for you. For example, if you have high blood pressure, it might not be an option.

- Wait at least two hours after eating before you sauna.

- If you shower before you sauna, you may sweat more; try it with and without showering first to see which you prefer.

- If this is your first experience with a sauna, stay in for just 10 minutes at a time, then follow with a cold shower and repeat a few times.

- Eating a piece of fruit after your sauna session helps replace potassium. Bananas are best.

- Drink plenty of water (at least two 8-ounce glasses) before and after your sauna.

● ● ● ● ● ● ● ● ● ● ● ● ● ● ● ● ● ● ●

Today the sauna is an integral strategy in purification programs, and I personally couldn't get by without taking a sauna at least three times a week. A sauna eliminates toxins including sodium, alcohol, and potentially carcinogenic heavy metals like cadmium, lead, and nickel. These toxins, which accumulate in our systems due to sluggish elimination processes, are removed from your body through perspiration. Sweating also works to treat cardiovascular conditions. In a study published in the *Journal of the American College of Cardiology,* 15 minutes in a sauna a day for 14 days improved the function of the endothelial cells lining the arteries by 40 percent. A sauna session will also reduce stress and give your skin an amazing glow. Perspiration is a beautiful thing.

REIKI: This ancient healing system uses energy to balance the body and mind. It works on several levels, from the physical and mental to the emotional and spiritual. It can reduce stress, thereby strengthening the body's natural immune system), aid in better sleep, and improve and maintain overall health. Its mental balancing capabilities also enhance learning, memory, and mental clarity. Mental health workers have attested to Reiki's ability to heal mental and emotional wounds. Susan Noss, MS, RD says, "In more severe situations, Reiki can help alleviate mood swings, fear, frustration, and even anger. Reiki can also strengthen and heal personal relationships." In turn, this treatment can bring a soothing calm and devotion to your week-long cleanse.

ACUPUNCTURE: Acupuncture is an ancient traditional Chinese medical procedure in which ultraskinny needles are inserted into points along "energy channels" called meridians, through which the life force of the human body flows. This helps unblock our clogged energy and in the process eases any discomfort that is a result of the blockage. There are hundreds of studies showing that acupuncture truly works. For example, the U.S. National Institutes of Health (NIH) reported a 44 percent average reduction in pain and a 40 percent improvement in mobility for arthritis sufferers after acupuncture treatments. Try not to be put off by the idea of being stuck with lots of needles. Even though it sounds like torture, most people report only a slight stinging sensation that lasts just a second when the needle first pricks the skin. After that, there's no pain, only gain.

MASSAGE: If you're preparing for the Cleanse, you probably don't need to be convinced there are accumulated toxins within you. Good news: Your body has its own natural method of detoxifying called the lymphatic system. Think of your lymphatic system as your body's sewer; it removes waste and purifies tissues through your lymph nodes.

HERE'S HOW IT WORKS: Lymph begins with plasma excreted from blood capillaries, carrying nutrients to your tissues and washing your cells to pick up metabolic waste and toxins. This now-contaminated fluid is absorbed into your microscopic lymph vessels and carried toward lymph nodes to be purified. After purification, lymph travels through progressively larger lymph vessels until it's returned to blood circulation through large veins in your neck. That's why during a cleanse the ideal type of massage treatment is a lymphatic drainage.

Lymphatic drainage massage is a gentle style of bodywork that mimics the movement of lymph vessels. Peripheral lymph vessels contract at a rate of 6 to 10 contractions per minute, so massage movements are repeated at the same slow rate. There's a rich bed of lymph capillaries immediately below your skin, so it isn't necessary to use deeper pressure to affect them. Lymph massage therapists use a light touch, less than nine ounces per square inch. Since lymph drains toward lymph nodes in the neck, armpits, and groin before traveling to the largest lymph vessels and back into the cardiovascular system, your therapist will massage your lymph nodes first, and then massage lymph toward the lymph nodes, before massaging your trunk and extremities. This kind of massage stimulates the reproduction and circulation of white blood cells and removes toxins from tissues, which are ultimately destroyed in your lymph nodes.

. . . .

DO-IT-YOURSELF LYMPHATIC DRAINAGE MASSAGE IN THREE EASY STEPS

If you don't have the finances to cover massages, or you want to increase their frequency without breaking your bank account, self-massage is a satisfying alternative. But don't cheat: Always complete your treatment by lying down and relaxing for at least 20 minutes.

- Beginning under your ears and using both hands, stroke down your neck and through to the hollows above your collarbone. Do this about 15 times.

- Now cross your arms over your chest. Press your index and middle fingers into the hollows above your collarbone and circle in opposite directions on each side. Repeat fifteen times.

- Next, raise one arm and massage your armpit in circles ten times. Repeat on the other side.

. . . .

ORGANIC SEA ALGAE WRAP: Most wrap treatments are pretty pricy, especially if they're offered in a fancy high-end spa, so check around for one that's not over the top. A good wrap will blend ingredients like algae with natural clay and an essential oil like lavender. Together these ingredients make for a powerful, detoxifying body wrap. Blue-green algae are the most nutrient-rich of all algae because they contain detoxifying chlorophyll and essential fatty acids that improve elasticity and stimulate your skin's natural healing. Meanwhile, clay draws out impurities while lavender's essential oil adds cleansing, balancing, and healing properties. The biggest benefit? Your lymphatic function will increase, which in turn will strengthen both your immune response and fat absorption. Some say it reduces cellulite, but there's no scientific evidence to support the claim.

SCALP TREATMENT: Sure, we think about our skin, but what about our heads? A good scalp treatment will offer gentle exfoliation to rid the scalp of impurities and provide the hair with energy and shine. A therapeutic shampoo and conditioner using all natural, patented, plant-derived ingredients adds nutrition, volume and shine. You can have it done at a spa for the ultimate in groovy sensations, or do it yourself.

MUD MASK: You can make this happen at home or go to a spa. But wherever your mask is enjoyed, be sure it's made of all natural mud (or clay). A mud mask detoxifies, rejuvenates and tones the skin. If home, after applying your own mask, lie on the sofa or bed, put your feet up on a pillow, and relax.

You'll find more at-home spa treatments during the cleanse week (page 81).

Step Six: Making the Dietary Transition

Things do not change; we change. —Henry David Thoreau

Change can knock your socks off and send you soaring barefoot and fancy free, but abrupt changes in diet can also throw you off center and flatten you to the ground. So for ultimate pleasure and optimum results, it's a better idea to ease into your new diet. This means adjusting your present one at least one week before you begin your Yoga-Body Cleanse.

If you don't prepare for your cleanse, you may experience more detox side effects such as nausea, moodiness, and bloating. You want to ease your metabolism into detoxing. You can do this by eliminating or at least cutting down on:

- Any food containing additives, preservatives, or chemicals

- Frozen, canned, or processed foods (opt for only fresh foods)

- Ice water and other cold drinks (stick to room temperature)

- Coffee and all caffeine products such as chocolate, black and green teas, and colas

- Alcohol

- Dairy products (milk, cheese, butter, ice cream, etc.)

- Eggs

- Sugar

- Meats

- Fried foods

It's important not to overeat during the days before your cleanse. Rather, consume light meals high in complex carbohydrates and moderate in protein and fat. Feasting right before you start the Yoga-Body Cleanse will force your body to compensate in metabolic extremes in terms of water, blood sugar levels, and heart rate. Besides, stuffing yourself can actually make you feel hungrier than if you ate lightly. Resist!

Here are some light but tasty predetoxing food choices:

- Fresh fruits like peaches, plums, apples, watermelon, banana, and papaya

- Green salad with vinaigrette or lemon dressing

- Steamed artichoke

- Lentil salad

- Hummus

Plus …

Be sure to add plenty of purified water to your daily routine. If you experience dark yellow or orange urine, dry mouth, constipation, joint pain, or dizziness, these are signs you might not be drinking enough water.

Chew slowly so your salivary glands can help your gastric juices do their job.

Step Seven: Set the Stage

In a perfect world, you would begin your purification in a secluded cabin atop a mountain with startling vistas, clean air, and a staff to attend to your every need, should you have any. Otherwise, solitude and peace would be your companions.

But I'm a realist and have had to juggle my cleansing diet with work and family. I'm confident that you can do it, too. What you'll need is a space all to yourself. Let the family know that you will be using the guest room, home office, laundry room, garage, or bathroom as your safe haven when you need to be alone to relax, meditate, or write down your thoughts. At work, use your lunch hours as a time to retreat into yourself. Don't be tempted to join a colleague for lunch, even if you're planning to sit across from her with a glass of water or a cup of tea. During this period in your life, choose to be alone as much as possible. Fellow cleansers have reported feeling closer to their spiritual centers and desire to pray. If this happens, go with your desire. Be conscious of a new self emerging; allow yourself to be led by inspiration. The most important point to remember is that this is your time. Leap with gusto into a new reality.

Write a Letter

To yourself! In it, write down a farewell to all the people, places, and behaviors that create toxins or limit your ability to stay focused and committed to your healing. You know what doesn't serve you, and it's usually something melodramatic.

Now write down all the reasons why you deserve to clean out your life and make it a positive, light-filled reality. While you're writing, don't forget to use your breath. The inhale will help you gather the strength and focus you need to conjure up your roadblocks. The deep, long exhale can help you release them and connect to the deeper, healthier parts of who you really are.

Make a Mantra Your Partner

A mantra is a sound, syllable, word, or group of words that is considered capable of creating transformation and healing on a deep level. "Om" may be the most famous one, but there are infinite mantras. You can make up your own or find one that resonates within your heart. You can repeat a mantra to yourself several times a day, whenever you find your mind wandering and want to change your thoughts, when you're driving, walking, or meditating. Here are a few options:

Om—According to the Dali Lama, "om" symbolizes the practitioner's impure body, speech, and mind; it also symbolizes the pure exalted body, speech, and mind of Buddha

Om Vajra Sattva Hum—Invokes a luminous balance

Om Namah Shivaya—Calls upon the great teacher within and all around

Om Hung Dun Durgaya Namaha—speaks to the great goddess Durga asking to open your heart and remove aspects in your life that lead to suffering

Om Mani Padme Hun — Said to be the most important mantra in Buddhism, the basic English translation of "om mani padme hum" is "om jewel in the lotus hum" or "praise to the jewel in the lotus."

Or just say "Ahh."

CHAPTER FOUR

7-DAY YOGA-BODY CLEANSE

Healing is a matter of time but it is sometimes also a matter of opportunity.

—Hippocrates

Now you're primed to dedicate seven days and seven nights to creating a new relationship with your body, spirit, and mind. As you'll experience, the Yoga-Body Cleanse not only rids your body of toxic elements and helps you look younger (and thinner) but it's also a full immersion process that enables you to be honest about where you are in your life right now and where you want to set new goals. You'll soon approach these areas openly because your body and mind will be in a receptive and relaxed state. The detox cleanse also guides you to let go of what no longer serves you. If you approach this project with a whole-hearted commitment and unshakeable confidence, it will be more easeful and, I promise, the rewards will not only be obvious, but enduring.

What to Expect

In this chapter you'll find seven days of meal plans (breakfast, lunch, dinner, and snacks), including food and juice recipes. Along with your daily menus, restorative yoga poses will be suggested each day. To help you stay focused and on a positive path, I'll also share affirmations. If you have your own, great! *Use* them. You'll also be offered over a dozen easy and natural detox beauty treatments from scrubs and facials, to aromatic and relaxing baths. Remember, you deserve to pamper yourself; these beauty treatments are easy to make and a pure pleasure to experience. You can create most of them just from ingredients found in your kitchen. Plus, I'll suggest activities from walking, meditating, and deep breathing to journal writing—all of which can deepen your awareness. Try to enjoy at least one or two of these elements daily. Keep in mind that the cleansing diet is not about denial; it's about discovery. It's not about courage; it's about letting go of discourage.

Day One

Morning

Time to begin!

1 Wake with the sunrise.

2 RECORD YOUR DREAMS: Sigmund Freud believed that
   dreams are a window into our unconscious, and several
   recent scientific studies indicate that he got it right.
   What's more, numerous cultures from Native Americans
   to Aborigines believe dreams are the key to our waking
   lives. One thing is certain: the memory of your dreams
   will fade quickly upon awakening. That's why you want
   as few impediments and distractions as possible between
   waking up and putting pen to paper. It's always best to
   write in your journal first thing in the morning, as soon
   as you wake up. Keep in mind that it's possible your
   dream life will grow more vivid as you detox.

Hint: *Make sure you have a bedside light that's easy to turn on.*

3 FOOT LANDING: Done writing in your journal? Before
   getting out of bed, try this reality check suggested by
   my chi gong teacher, Sat Hon. Simply remember which
   foot, left or right, lands on the floor first when you get
   out of bed. You may be surprised how this be-here-now
   exercise is tough to carry out. As the days of your cleanse
   move behind you, and you connect more consciously to
   the moment you're in, odds are this exercise will become
   second nature and you'll begin your day with sharpened
   awareness of the present.

4 Recite *your* affirmation or use this: *"Loving myself heals my life. I nourish my mind, body, and soul."*

5 Scrape your tongue.

6 Drink an 8-ounce glass of water with lemon. It's best if the water is hot.

· ·

THE BEAUTY OF HOT LEMON WATER

This drink will do more than quench your thirst and hydrate your body. It also flushes out the liver and bumps up mineral absorption. Cold beverages do the opposite: They cool digestion and can slow it down, so avoid chilly liquids while cleansing.

· ·

7 Soak one cup of mung (split yellow) beans to prepare for Kitchari (page 86).

8 YOGA: Three-minute shoulder stretch (Urdhva Hastansana)

With your bare feet firmly planted on the ground, interlace your fingers and raise your arms above your head with your palms facing upward. Keep your arms in line with your ears while you look straight ahead and relax your shoulder blades down your back. Hold for five full breaths through your nose. Let your arms fall down to your sides, roll your shoulders backward and forward a few times, then repeat the stretch three more times, holding for five full breaths.

9 MEDITATION/MANTRA: Sit in a comfortable position for at least 15 minutes. You may want to increase the time you spend in meditation as your body detoxes. Since being concerned about time can be distracting, you may also find it helps to simply set a timer and let the clock be concerned about how long you have to meditate. Try setting a timer on your smartphone to a soothing tone.

• •

FIRST TIME MEDITATING? THREE SIMPLE STEPS

1 Sit on a cushion or a straight-backed chair. You don't have to adopt any unusual postures. The important thing is to keep your back straight. Relax your arms and legs. They don't need to be in any special position, either.

2 Let your attention rest on the flow of your breath. Listen to it, follow it, but make no judgments about it. Find a focus to settle your mind. Or, try reciting your mantra. Counting your breath from 1 through 10 also works. Each time you realize you've lost track begin again at 1.

3 Once you've trained your mind to focus on just one thing at a time, the next step is to focus on nothing at all, essentially "clearing" your mind. This requires discipline but it's the true goal of meditation. After anchoring on a single point (as described above), you can either cast it away or observe it impartially and let it come and then go, without labeling it as "good" or "bad." Take the same approach to any thoughts which return to your mind until silence perseveres.

• •

10 PREPARE A POT OF KITCHARI: Kitchari is the traditional dish to consume while on an Ayurvedic-based cleansing diet. It's a mix of rice, split yellow mung beans, and optionally, clarified butter (ghee). Spices and seasonal vegetables are also optional. Since kitchari is so easy to digest, it sparks your metabolic system to burn off old toxins while creating a healthful balance.

KITCHARI
PREP TIME: About 1 hour

1 cup split yellow mung beans
(not whole dal)

½ cup white basmati rice

1 tablespoon finely minced fresh ginger root

1 teaspoon black mustard seeds

1 teaspoon ground cumin

1 teaspoon ground turmeric powder

½ teaspoon coriander powder

½ teaspoon fennel seeds

½ teaspoon fenugreek seeds

3 bay leaves

½ teaspoon sea salt, plus more for serving

7 to 10 cups water

Seasonal vegetables *(optional)*

Pat of ghee *(optional)*

Cilantro, to serve *(optional)*

Wash the split yellow mung beans and rice together in a fine-mesh sieve until the water runs clear. Heat a large pot over a medium heat and then add all the spices and dry roast for few minutes. This dry-roasting will enhance the flavor. Add the water and bring to a boil for 10 minutes. If you prefer your kitchari to have consistency of oatmeal rather than soup, use the lesser quantity of liquid. Turn the heat to low, cover, and continue to cook for about 20 minutes, until all the water is absorbed. Add the veggies and cook for about another 20 minutes, until the beans and rice become soft. Stir in a pat of ghee for added creaminess, if desired. If you like, garnish with cilantro leaves just before serving. Add sea salt to taste.

11 BREAKFAST: Bowl of kitchari. Choose a single-size serving bowl and use it each time you enjoy your kitchari. Measure the amount you will be eating by cupping your hands together as if you were receiving something precious in it. In Sanskrit this is called *anjali*; it's the perfect size for one serving.

A monk came to Joshu and asked,
"What is the meaning of Zen?"
The Master replied, "Have you eaten your breakfast?"
"Yes," said the monk. "I have eaten."
"Then wash your bowl," said Joshu.
At that instant the monk was enlightened.

  —from *The Little Book of Zen Wisdom*, compiled by Jon Baldock

---

Whenever you're going to consume a meal during your cleanse, first find a quiet place that offers you peace and solitude; perhaps say a prayer of gratitude before eating. Take slow and mindful spoonfuls as you eat.

12 SNACK: Choose from

✿ Organic flaxseed and brown rice crackers

✿ Homemade popcorn with ghee and sea salt

✿ Seaweed snacks

✿ Fruit: fresh, in-season, but limit quantity

✿ Seeds and nuts

✿ Great Green Juice 1

GREAT GREEN JUICE 1

½ head celery
6 leaves beet greens
1 small cucumber
2 tablespoons fresh lemon juice

Chop the ingredients into pieces small enough for either your blender blade to crush easily or to fit into the feeder of your juicer. Start with the celery and end with the cucumber. Stir in the lemon juice and add as much water as needed to make your 16-ounce serving.

Afternoon

1 LUNCH: If you want to eat any raw food, it's recommended to eat it for lunch, rather than breakfast or dinner. If not, enjoy a simple serving of kitchari (page 86).

2 How about a walk?

3   SNACK: Great Green Juice 1 (page 88)

4   YOGA: Supported Legs Up the Wall (Salama Vipariti Karani)

Set your mat vertically against a wall. Fold a blanket to the size of a bed pillow; then fold it again two-thirds of the way down so you have a thinner edge for your neck and head. Raise your legs against the wall and lower yourself gently so that your middle and upper back are on your mat and your head and neck are on the blanket. Rest your hands by your side and close your eyes. Give yourself 20 minutes to relax.

Evening

1   DINNER: Enjoy a bowl of Kitchari (page 86). If you're in the mood, add cooked dark green vegetables like spinach, kale, or dandelion greens.

2   PAMPER BEFORE BED: Shower and scrub. Oil your body from head (including scalp) to toes and soles with room temperature olive oil or flaxseed oil. Step carefully into a warm shower and let the water gently wash over you. Using a shower brush or loofah, scrub your body vigorously and thoroughly. Give attention under your breasts, armpits, stomach, inner thighs, butt, legs, and feet. If you've poured oil on your scalp, shampoo it out with an all-natural organic product. Be careful stepping out of the shower in case your feet are still oily. Pat yourself dry with a fluffy towel and feel the texture of your new supple, baby-soft skin. You can experience a shower scrub every evening or alternate with different

bathing activities. Beginning Day Two, add an additional pampering treatment. You deserve it.

3 EASE INTO SLEEP: While your body is adjusting to its new condition, sleep may be elusive. To coax it into slumber, be sure to shut off all electronics an hour before going to bed. Read poetry or inspirational books. Definitely avoid thrillers! You're life is thrilling enough. Perhaps you want to write in your journal? In any case, before shutting your eyes, make an intention to remember your dreams.

Day Two

Morning

1 Wake with the sunrise.

2 Record your dreams.

3 Pay attention to which foot lands on the floor when stepping out of bed.

4 Recite *your* affirmation. Or try this one: *"There is within each of us the possibility of magnificence."* —Marianne Williamson

5 Scrape your tongue.

6 Enjoy a cup of hot water with lemon.

7 THREE-MINUTE YOGA: Standing Forward Bend (Uttanasana)

Exhale and fold forward over your legs into a forward bend. If your hamstrings feel a little tight at first, bend your knees so that you can release your spine. Let your head hang heavy. Slowly straighten the legs if you like, but keep the head hanging. Your feet can be touching or be hips' distance apart, whichever feels better. Slowly roll up with bent knees, one vertebra at a time. Repeat three times. Take your time.

8 MEDITATION

9 BREAKFAST: Choose from

🌿 Kitchari (page 86)

🌿 Steel-cut oatmeal with sliced apple and seeds of choice

10 When stress or a difficult situation arises during the day, imagine you're standing in a tree house looking down at it—and remember to breathe deeply.

11 SNACK: Choose from

🌿 Organic flaxseed and brown rice crackers

🌿 Homemade popcorn with ghee and sea salt

🌿 Seaweed snacks

🌿 Fruit: fresh, in-season, but limit quantity

🌿 Seeds and nuts

🌿 Great Green Juice 2

GREAT GREEN JUICE 2

5 leaves romaine lettuce
1 cucumber
3 celery ribs
2 handfuls blueberries (if in season)
½ Granny Smith apple
¼ lemon

Make sure you wash your ingredients before you pass them through the juicer and core the apple. You might want to leave a bit of the lemon rind on for flavor.

Afternoon

1   LUNCH: Choose from

    ✤   Bowl of Kitchari (page 86)

    ✤   Simple green salad with freshly squeezed lemon or
       lime juice as dressing

    ✤   Cooked green leafy vegetables with quinoa

2   How about writing in your journal?

3   SNACK: Great Green Juice 2 (page 92)

4   YOGA: Child's Pose (Balasana)

Easing your body into child's pose allows for a gentle stretch
in the hips and legs, while relieving stress in the back and
neck. Move into child's pose by kneeling on the floor with
your big toes touching. Sit back on your heels and position
your knees hip-width apart. On an exhale, bend forward
at the waist and bring your forehead down to the floor.
Lengthen your spine by extending your head and tailbone
away from one another. Lay your hands at your sides with
your hands resting near your feet. Hold for as long as it feels
comforting.

Evening

1   DINNER: Choose from

    ✤   Bowl of Kitchari (page 86)

    ✤   Cooked greens and a grain, such as buckwheat

2   Create a tranquil home spa where you can unwind and rejuvenate in your bathroom. It's easy to create and the payoff is immeasurable. Between 7:00 and 8:00 p.m., at least three times a week, I retreat to my personal "sanctum sanitarium." My family knows that unless it's an emergency, I am to be left alone, undisturbed. Let the rich and famous pay extravagant sums to be buffed and smoothed in a luxury spa. I have it in my own home and on my own time. And so can you. Oh, I can hear you protesting, "It's impossible to take all this time for myself!" Consider your spa sessions an indispensable element in your detoxing program.

You'll want to have a few of these soothing essentials on hand:

- ❧ Natural beeswax candles/matches
- ❧ Body buffer for dry brushing
- ❧ Pumice stone
- ❧ Natural botanic shampoo
- ❧ Music system with your favorite music
- ❧ Spring water
- ❧ Thick, soft bath towel
- ❧ Cozy robe

Set the stage. Turn on your music with the volume on low and place your candles strategically so their reflection flickers on the water. Slowly undress while watching yourself in the mirror. Think positive thoughts about your body. If you find yourself dwelling on a body part you don't like, tell yourself,

"That's not the whole picture of my being." And affirm: *"Although my body is the temple of my soul, it is the true nature of my soul that projects outward."* Since your time is precious, opt for the treatment that suits your particular need for the day.

3 CHOOSE ONE BATHING TREATMENT:

DETOXING AROMATHERAPY BATH: Cut the leg from a clean pair of panty hose; fill with 1 tablespoon each of dried chamomile and rosemary and add 4 drops for lavender oil. Knot one end of the panty hose to form a sachet, then tie it under the faucet so that the very warm water runs through. Fill the tub and soak for 30 minutes, sipping from your bottle of spring water. The herbs have a calming effect while the water temperature raises body heat and eliminates impurities.

AROMA BATH: Add 15 to 30 drops essential oil of choice (lavender is the most relaxing!) to 1 ounce olive oil, flaxseed oil, or other oil of choice. Fill a small-mouth jar with the oil. Add the essential oils drop by drop, cap the jar with a tight-fitting lid and shake well. Use 1-2 teaspoons of oil per bath.

4 EASE INTO SLEEP: Shut down electronics. Make an intention to remember your dreams.

Day Three

Morning

1 Wake with the sunrise.

2 Record your dreams.

3 Pay attention to which foot lands on the floor when stepping out of bed.

4 Recite *your* affirmation. Or try this one: Every cell in my body vibrates with energy and health.

5 Scrape your tongue.

6 Enjoy a cup of hot water with lemon.

7 YOGA: Spinal Twist (Ardha Matsyandrasana)

Spinal twists help improve digestion, add flexibility to the spine, and lessen back pain. Sit with your legs straight out in front of you; lengthen through your heels. Pull the flesh away from your sitz bones and press them into the earth. Bend your right knee and place your right foot on the opposite side of the left knee. Continue lengthening the left foot, keeping it flexed. Check in with your alignment. Press through the sitz bones. Inhale up the front side of the body lifting the pelvic floor, diaphragm, and sternum, tuck the chin, and lengthen through the crown of the head. Relax your lower back. Relax your face, the jaw, the space between the eyebrows. Now you're ready to twist. Inhale as you raise and extend your right hand in front of you. Gaze at your fingertips. Exhale and twist to the right. Work with your breath: Inhale then lengthen. Exhale then twist. When you're as far as your body wants to go, place your hand to the earth toward your sacrum. Now continue twisting. Even twist the eyes looking to the corner of the room. Breathe. When you are ready to release, inhale the arm up and release as slowly as you entered the twist. Prepare for the opposite side by alternating your legs.

8   MEDITATION

9   BREAKFAST: Choose from a bowl of

- ❧ Kitchari (page 86)

- ❧ Steel-cut oatmeal with sliced apple and seeds of choice

- ❧ Homemade Breakfast Cereal

HOMEMADE BREAKFAST CEREAL

1 cup purified water
Pinch of salt
¼ cup buckwheat groats

In a small saucepan, bring the water and salt to a boil over high heat. Stir in the buckwheat and return to a boil. Reduce the heat to low and simmer, uncovered, for 10 minutes or until thickened. Stir frequently.

10 SNACK: Choose from

- ❧ Organic flaxseed and brown rice crackers

- ❧ Homemade popcorn with ghee and sea salt

- ❧ Seaweed snacks

- ❧ Fruit: fresh, in-season, but limit quantity

- 🌿 Seeds and nuts
- 🌿 Great Green Juice 3 (page 98)

GREAT GREEN JUICE 3

Handful of spinach

3 medium stalks of kale

2 granny smith apples

½ large cucumber

Small handful of parsley *(remove the long stems)*

1 lemon

Wash all the ingredients. Trim most of the peel from the lemon and quarter and core the apples. Cut the cucumber into pieces that either your juicer or blender will accept. After juicing, scrape off the foam.

Afternoon

1   LUNCH: Choose from

- 🌿 Bowl of Kitchari (page 86)
- 🌿 Simple green salad with freshly squeezed lemon or lime juice as dressing
- 🌿 Cooked green leafy vegetables with quinoa
- 🌿 Cold Spinach Soup (page 99)

COLD SPINACH SOUP

2 cups fresh spinach

1 cup purified water

1 celery stalk chopped

2 tablespoons fresh lemon juice

Puree all the ingredients in a blender until it's the consistency you enjoy.

2   Feeling a spark of creativity? Try writing a haiku, a descriptive poem of 17 syllables and composed of three lines or word groups, usually unrhymed:

Line #1: five syllables

Line #2: seven syllables

Line #3: five syllables

Here's an example written by Basho, a Zen Buddhist monk:

> on a bare branch
> a crow has alighted
> autumn evening.

3   SNACK: Great Green Juice 3 (page 98)

4   YOGA: Supine Bound Angle Pose (Baddha Konasana)

Lie on your back, or over a bolster (a cushion works too), with your knees bent and your feet touching the floor. Slowly open your knees out wide, so that the soles of your feet are touching. Relax for at least five full minutes with eyes closed. When you're ready to stand, roll to your right side, then to knees, then upright.

Evening

1. DINNER: Choose from

   ꧁ Bowl of Kitchari (page 86)

   ꧁ Steamed greens and grain

   ꧁ Roasted Beets (page 100)

ROASTED BEETS

4 to 6 beets
1 pinch fresh rosemary
1 pinch fresh or dried thyme
2 small cloves garlic
Sea salt, to taste
3 tablespoons olive oil

Preheat the oven to 350°F. Clean the dirt from the beets and trim at both ends. Place foil on a cookie sheet or pan, then place the beets on top along with garlic. Drizzle olive oil and sprinkle on rosemary, thyme, whole cloves of garlic, and salt. Add one cup of water to the pan before covering tightly with foil. Roast in the oven for 45 minutes or until the beets are tender. Once the roasted beets are cooled enough to touch, gently squeeze the beet to break open the skin and peel off.

2 PAMPERING AND BATHING TREATMENTS: Choose one or two

   ꧁ Buff and scrub shower

SUPER STRESS-BUSTING BATH: Brew one cup of chamomile tea and add 10 drops of lavender oil. Add to the bath. While you're soaking, practice deep breathing: Inhale and exhale slowly, focusing on your breath.

SOOTHING HAND SOAK: Soak your hands in warm olive oil and follow with this healing massage: Mix two parts of cooked oatmeal with equal amounts of milk and two drops of rose water. Rub the mixture on your hands for several minutes; then rinse.

SIMPLE ANTIOXIDANT MASK: Steam one large carrot, and mash it thoroughly. To achieve a pasty consistency, add a small amount of purified water. Apply to your face for 10 minutes, then rinse off.

3   EASE INTO SLEEP: Shut down electronics, etc. Make an intention to remember your dreams. Visualize a river. Quietly watch the beautiful, flowing water and see yourself and your life floating smoothly.

Day Four

Morning

1   Wake with the sunrise.

2   Record your dreams.

3   Pay attention to which foot lands first on the floor when stepping out of bed.

4   Recite *your* affirmation. Or try this one: *"I choose love, joy, and freedom, open my heart, and allow wonderful things to flow into my life."*

5   Scrape your tongue.

6   Enjoy a cup of hot water with lemon.

7   YOGA: Happy Baby Pose (Ananda Balasana)

Lie on your back and bend your knees, hugging them in toward your chest. Then take the outer edges of your feet in your hands, reaching your knees toward your armpits. (If this is too much, take your hands to the back of your thighs.) Rock softly from left to right if that feels nice; stay here for 10 deep breaths.

8   MEDITATION

9   BREAKFAST: Choose from a bowl of

   ❧ Kitchari (page 86)

- 🌿 Steel-cut oatmeal with sliced apple and seeds of choice
- 🌿 Homemade Breakfast Cereal (page 97)

Gratitude research is beginning to suggest that feelings of thankfulness have tremendous positive value in helping people cope with daily problems, especially stress.

— University of California Davis psychology professor Robert Emmons

---

10 SNACK: Choose from

- 🌿 Organic flaxseed and brown rice crackers
- 🌿 Homemade popcorn with ghee and sea salt
- 🌿 Seaweed snacks
- 🌿 Fruit: fresh, in-season, but limit your fruits.
- 🌿 Seeds and nuts
- 🌿 Great Green Juice 4 (page 103)

GREAT GREEN JUICE 4

Handful of spinach
2 medium carrots
1 lime
¼ pineapple
Pinch of cayenne (optional)

Wash spinach and carrots. Cut the peel from lime. Run ingredients through blender and juicer.

Afternoon

11 LUNCH: Choose from

- 🌱 Bowl of Kitchari (page 86)

- 🌱 Simple green salad with freshly squeezed lemon or lime juice as dressing

- 🌱 Cooked green leafy vegetables with quinoa

- 🌱 Cold Spinach Soup (page 99)

Remember to eat slowly and consciously!

12 Your mind is quieting and you can probably notice the small feelings that ordinarily get drowned out. Cry! Laugh! Experience regrets! Applaud your accomplishments! Feel the joy!

13 SNACK: Great Green Juice 4 (page 103)

14 YOGA: Corpse Pose (Savasana) with Leg Support

While seated with your legs long in front of you and just a bit apart, roll up a blanket and place it under your knees. Lie down on your back, allowing your legs to separate with your feet about hip-distance apart and your arms to relax on either side of you. Breathe here for at least 20 deep breaths or as long as you like.

Evening

1 DINNER: Choose from

- 🌿 Bowl of Kitchari (page 86)

- 🌿 Steamed greens and grain

- 🌿 Roasted Beets (page 100)

2 BATHING TREATMENTS: Choose one

- 🌿 Buff and scrub shower

- 🌿 Super stress-busting bath (page 100)

- 🌿 Muscle-relaxing bath (page 159)

3 PAMPERING: Choose one or two

- 🌿 Soothing hand soak (page 101)

- 🌿 Simple antioxidant mask (page 101)

YOGURT COOLING MASK: Mix 3 teaspoons of plain organic yogurt and 3 tablespoons of honey, which locks in moisture. Smooth onto your clean skin and leave on for 15 minutes. Remove with cool spring water. Now apply pure aloe vera juice with a cotton ball. Aloe vera not only cleanses your skin but also heals and detoxifies it.

4 EASE INTO SLEEP: Shut down electronics, etc. Make an intention to remember your dreams.

No more words. In the name of this place we drink in with our breathing, stay quiet like a flower. So the nightbirds will start singing. —Rumi, *Night and Sleep*

Day Five

Morning

Now that you're on Day Five of your 7-Day Yoga-Body Cleanse, your body and spirit is ripe to ease into a deeper awareness. To help facilitate this transition, today you'll drink *only* fresh green juices and smoothies. Notice how your body and awareness feels ready for this shift.

During juice days, expend less energy. Relax more. Watch your thoughts come and go.

---

1   Wake with the sunrise.

2   Record your dreams.

3   Pay attention to which foot lands first on the floor when stepping out of bed.

4   Recite *your* affirmation. Or try this one: *"I choose to live my life the way that makes me happy and I am free."*

5   Scrape your tongue.

6   Enjoy a cup of hot water with lemon.

7   YOGA: Thread the Needle Pose (variation on Eka Pada Rajakapotasana)

From all fours, reach your right arm underneath your body, allowing your right shoulder and temple to release to the ground. Your left hand can stay where it is, or crawl a bit to the right over your head. Breathe here for 10 deep breaths; then repeat on the other side.

8 MEDITATION

9 BREAKFAST: Your choice of Great Green Juice 1, 2, or 3 (pages 88, 92, and 98).

10 SNACK: Apple Beet Juice

APPLE BEET JUICE

1½ Granny Smith apples
3 small red beets
1 inch piece of ginger

Wash all your ingredients. Cut the apple and beet so they will fit through the juicer or mush with the blender's blades. Scrape off the foam.

Afternoon

1 LUNCH: Your choice of Great Green Juice 1, 2, or 3 (pages 88, 92, and 98). Sip slowly and feel the gratitude.

2 ALTERNATE DETOXING BREATHS: Sit comfortably in a straight-backed chair. Close the right nostril by pinching it, and breathe in slowly through the left. When you have taken a full breath, close both nostrils for as long as is comfortable; then, keeping the left nostril closed, exhale slowly through the right. Now inhale through the right nostril, hold, and exhale through the left. Try this up to 10 times.

3   SNACK: Your choice of Great Green Juice 1, 2, or 3 (pages 88, 92, and 98). Sip slowly and feel the gratitude.

4   YOGA: Pigeon Pose (Eka Pada Rajakapotasana)

Sweep your right shin toward the front of your mat, right knee toward your right wrist, and right ankle toward your left wrist. (If your right hip is elevated, set a rolled blanket or firm pillow underneath it.) Crawl your hands forward until your head is on the ground (or prop your head up with soft blocks or blankets), and breathe here for 10 deep breaths. Repeat on the left side.

Evening

1   DINNER: Great Green Juice 4 (page 103)

2   BATHING TREATMENTS: Muscle relaxing bath (page 159)

3   PAMPERING

MIGHTY MOISTURIZER: In India women keep their complexions glowing with rose water sprayed lightly on the face and allowed to dry, followed with a bit of ghee (clarified butter), which moisturizes and protects the skin. Wear this lovely cream to bed.

4   EASE INTO SLEEP: Shut down electronics, etc. Make an intention to remember your dreams.

Sleep is the best meditation.   — Dalai Lama

Day Six

Today you'll continue with a mostly juice menu. If you were experiencing feelings of hunger, they probably lessened by yesterday. Remember to stay hydrated by drinking plenty of water.

Morning

1 Wake with the sunrise.

2 Record your dreams.

3 Pay attention to which foot lands first on the floor when stepping out of bed. (Do you have this down pat, yet?)

4 Recite *your* affirmation. Or try this one: *"I embrace the rhythm and the flowing of my own heart."*

5 Scrape your tongue.

6 Enjoy a cup of hot water with lemon.

7 YOGA: Puppy Pose (Uttana Shishosana)

This is a variation of child's pose with a heart–opening effect. Come onto all fours. See that your shoulders are over your wrists and your hips are over your knees. Walk your hands forward a few inches and curl your toes under. As you exhale, move your buttocks to the floor or a blanket, and let your neck relax. Keep a slight curve in your lower back. To feel a nice long stretch in your spine, press the hands down and stretch through the arms while pulling your hips back toward your heels. Breathe into your back, feeling the spine lengthen in both directions. Hold for 30 seconds to a minute, then release your buttocks down onto your heels.

8 MEDITATION

• • • • • • • • • • • • • • • • • • • •

CHECK IT OUT:

- Are your senses more alive?
- Does your body feel lithe and strong?
- Look in the mirror — Is a bright-eyed youthful reflection returning your gaze?
- Are friends and acquaintances telling you how great you look or wondering "what's different?"
- Are your perceptions more powerful?

• • • • • • • • • • • • • • • • • • • •

9 BREAKFAST: Your choice of Great Green Juice 1, 2, 3, or 4 (pages 88, 92, 98, and 103).

10 SNACK: Choose from

    🌿 Apple Beet Juice (page 107)

    🌿 Mint Lemonade (page 111)

MINT LEMONADE

2 cups boiled water
1 herbal mint tea bag
Juice of one lemon
1 tablespoon of real maple syrup
(optional)

Stir together all ingredients. Refrigerate until cold.

Afternoon

1 LUNCH: Your choice of Great Green Juice 1, 2, 3, or 4 (pages 88, 92, 98, and 103).

As you open to higher realms of peace and love, you see that the key to these levels of reality is forgiveness. Who can you open your heart to forgive?

2 RELAXING BREATH: Sit in a chair with your back straight. Place the tip of your tongue against the ridge of tissue

just behind your upper front teeth, and keep it there through the entire exercise. You will be exhaling through your mouth around your tongue. Exhale completely through your mouth, making a whoosh sound. Close your mouth and inhale quietly through your nose to a mental count of four. Hold your breath for a count of seven. Exhale completely through your mouth, making a whoosh sound to a count of eight. This is one breath. Now inhale again and repeat the cycle three more times for a total of four breaths.

3 SNACK: Your choice of Great Green Juice 1, 2, 3, or 4 (pages 88, 92, 98, and 103).

4 YOGA: Cat Pose (Marjaryasana)

The cat pose soothes and stretches the lower back, relieving stress while gently massaging the spine. Get on your hands and knees on your mat. Keep your hands directly beneath your shoulders and your knees directly beneath your hips. Spread your fingers. Your middle finger should be facing forward. Gaze at the floor. Breathe in deeply. On an exhale, gently pull your abdominal muscles backward toward your spine. Tuck your tailbone down and under. Gently contract your glutes. Release by sitting backward on your heels with your torso upright. Try this 10 times.

Evening

1 DINNER: Bowl of Kitchari (page 86)

2 BATHING TREATMENTS: Shower and scrub

3 PAMPERING

BE KIND TO YOUR FEET: Soak your feet in warm water and honey for ten minutes. This will help to get rid of the dryness and your feet will become soft and supple. Gently massage your feet and then wash them with lukewarm water.

Verses 13:14–17, Jesus instructs his disciples: *"If I then, your Lord and Teacher, have washed your feet, you also ought to wash one another's feet."*

4 EASE INTO SLEEP: Shut down electronics, etc. Make an intention to remember your dreams.

To sleep, perchance to dream.   — William Shakespeare, *Hamlet*

Day Seven

Morning

Congratulations! You've reached your final day of the Yoga–Body Cleanse! You will find that tasks and projects that took you days to muddle through will be done without hesitation. With a clear mind and body, your creativity flows unbridled and allows you to accomplish your goals. You'll be so efficient you may be wondering "What next?" Hey, that's up to you.

1   Wake with the sunrise.

2   Record your dreams.

3   Pay attention to which foot lands first on the floor when stepping out of bed. (By now this is probably second nature!)

4   Recite *your* affirmation. Or try this one: *"I let go of a life without goals and replace it with a destiny of success and grand achievement."*

5   Scrape your tongue.

6   Enjoy a cup of hot water with lemon.

7   YOGA: Bridge Pose (Setu Bandha Sarvangasana)

This pose provides gentle stretching of the back and legs while alleviating stress and tension. The pose can reduce anxiety, fatigue, backaches, headaches, and insomnia, and is even thought to be therapeutic for high blood pressure. Lie down facing upward on your mat. Take a few deep breaths to get grounded and relaxed. Bend your knees, plant your feet flat on the floor, and make sure the knees are hips-distance apart. As you push your pelvis up and forward, your knees should be directly over your heels. Keep your arms extended on either side of your body with palms facing down. Release your butt yet be sure to keep your thighs strong and engaged in order to get those hips even higher. When you're coming out of bridge pose, release your clasped hands and slowly bring your body back to the ground. Repeat three times, and after the series, bring your knees toward your chest for a squeeze.

8 MEDITATION

9 BREAKFAST: Choose from

- ❀ Kitachri (page 86)
- ❀ Steel-cut oatmeal with sliced apple and seeds of choice

10 SNACK: Choose from

- ❀ Organic flaxseed and brown rice crackers
- ❀ Homemade popcorn with ghee and sea salt
- ❀ Seaweed snacks
- ❀ Fruit: fresh, in-season, but limit your fruits
- ❀ Seeds and nuts
- ❀ Your choice of Great Green Juice 1, 2, 3, or 4 (pages 88, 92, 98, and 103).

Afternoon

1   LUNCH: Choose from

    🌿 Bowl of Kitchari (page 86)

    🌿 Simple green salad with freshly squeezed lemon or lime juice as dressing

    🌿 Cooked green leafy vegetables with quinoa

    🌿 Cold Spinach Soup (page 99)

Happiness expands within me. It lightens my life and touches everyone I meet.

---

2   JOURNAL WRITING: You may or may not decide to continue writing in your journal, but make this entry even if it's your last. You're in a wildly open and accepting space now, cleared of toxins, relieved of stressed, and hopefully your heart has opened. Write down your thoughts so in the future you can return to your journal and recall your amazing journey.

3   SNACK: Your choice of Great Green Juice 1, 2, 3, or 4 (pages 88, 92, 98, and 103).

14 YOGA: Corpse Pose (Savasana)

Most yoga practices end with several minutes spent in Savasana. This pose is a perfect way to honor all your efforts. Plus, it will put your body completely at ease, emphasizing total relaxation. Savasana can trigger the body's "relaxation response," a state of deep rest that slows the breathing and lowers the blood pressure while quieting the nervous system. On your back, the arms and legs are spread at about 45 degrees, the eyes are closed. Let your whole body is relax onto the floor or mat with an awareness of your chest and abdomen rising and falling with each breath. Scan all parts of your body for muscular tension of any kind, and consciously release if any are found. Feel free to stay in this relaxed position for as long as you like.

Evening

1   Dinner: Choose from

  ❧ Bowl of Kitchari (page 86) with steamed vegetables

  ❧ Cooked greens and grain

2   BATHING TREATMENTS

  ❧ Shower and scrub

3   PAMPERING

BANANA FACIAL CREAM: Mash half of a ripe banana until creamy. Apply to your face and leave for 15 to 20 minutes. Rinse with warm water and cold water to close pores. Pat dry.

SMOOTH HANDS: Mix 1 ounce ground almonds, 1 teaspoon clear honey, 2 teaspoons olive oil, and 1 teaspoon of lemon juice into a thick paste. Rub a heaping teaspoon all over the hands for two to three minutes and rinse off.

4 EASE INTO SLEEP: Shut down electronics, etc. Make an intention to remember your dreams.

Even a soul submerged in sleep is hard at work and helps make something of the world.   —Heraclitus, *Fragments*

CHAPTER FIVE

REST! RESTORE! RENEWAL!

True happiness comes from the joy of deeds well done, the zest of creating things new.

— Antoine de Saint-Exupery

You've just spent a week devoting your time and focus to cleaning out your body, revitalizing your spirit, and connecting to your power. Lots of folks who follow the 7-Day Yoga–Body Cleanse report they've never felt better in their lives. That's saying a lot, but I know what they mean. Honestly? I feel awesome after I cleanse. If you're also sailing under a bright sun on a tranquil sea, join the crew. I suspect these days, worries are drifting away rather than taking hold; you're also finding yourself relying more on your intuition to point you in the right direction. There's a good chance you have more energy, glowing skin, a dynamic digestive system, and a real sense of drive and motivation. Might you also be fitting into your smaller–sized jeans? Hallelujah!

Will your post-detox, blissed-out glow last forever? Well, how long it lasts mostly depends on you. You're more likely to crash a lot quicker and harder if you decide to celebrate the end of your week with a few drinks, fried food, and/or lots of sweets and processed foods; or if you're opting to jump back into old emotional patterns or hanging out with friends who are needy sponges. The good news? Crashing is avoidable.

In this chapter you'll be offered plenty of simple recipes for easy-to-digest foods that can keep you on course. I'll slowly reintroduce dairy as well as reasonable sweets back into your diet. But whatever you do or don't decide to eat, keep it simple and monitor your portions. You'll likely need considerably less food to feel full now. Don't push yourself to eat more! Also, try to continue some of your healthy habits, particularly eating in a peaceful environment. Take time to appreciate how good food tastes after not eating a lot.

You'll also find plenty of soul-enriching exercises in this chapter, as well as additional pampering treatments, yoga poses, and meditative techniques to keep you in a deep, whole place. But first take the "How Renewed Are You?" and discover just how far you've come and where you need to place a bit more healing energy and continue your good progress.

I know of no more encouraging fact than the unquestionable ability of man to elevate his life by conscious endeavor.
— Henry David Thoreau

How Renewed Are You?

Answer each question with Never, Occasionally, or Frequently.

PART ONE: YOUR SPIRIT

1 I wake in the morning excited about the day.
   O Never   O Occasionally   O Frequently

2 I remember many dreams and write them down.
   O Never   O Occasionally   O Frequently

3 I'm less likely to dwell on negative thoughts.
   O Never   O Occasionally   O Frequently

4 I remind myself to be in the moment.
   O Never   O Occasionally   O Frequently

5 I'm practicing forgiveness.
   O Never   O Occasionally   O Frequently

6 I feel blessed to be alive.
   O Never   O Occasionally   O Frequently

7 I've had lots of creative ideas lately.
   O Never   O Occasionally   O Frequently

8 I don't get as angry or frustrated as I did before the cleanse.
   O Never   O Occasionally   O Frequently

9 My heart feels more open to compassion and less to judgment.
   O Never   O Occasionally   O Frequently

10 I'm trusting my intuition.
   O Never   O Occasionally   O Frequently

PART TWO: YOUR BODY

1 I sleep through the night.
   O Never   O Occasionally   O Frequently

2 I've either given up coffee or drink less of it.
   O Never   O Occasionally   O Frequently

3 I have lots more energy than before my cleanse.
   O Never   O Occasionally   O Frequently

4 I have a daily yoga and/or meditation practice.
   O Never   O Occasionally   O Frequently

5 I spend less time sitting on the couch and watching television.
   O Never   O Occasionally   O Frequently

6 I crave fewer sweets.
   O Never   O Occasionally   O Frequently

7 In general, I eat less.
   O Never   O Occasionally   O Frequently

8 When I can, I'll walk or bike somewhere rather than drive.
   O Never   O Occasionally   O Frequently

9 I have much more energy.
   O Never   O Occasionally   O Frequently

10 I'm tuned into my body's needs.
   O Never   O Occasionally   O Frequently

PART THREE: YOUR EMOTIONS

1   I'm more likely to say "no" if I know something is going to stress me out.
    O Never   O Occasionally   O Frequently

2   I spend less time with, or I've let go of, toxic relationships.
    O Never   O Occasionally   O Frequently

3   Moods come and go but I don't get stuck in any for long.
    O Never   O Occasionally   O Frequently

4   I'm experiencing frequent spontaneous feelings of gratitude.
    O Never   O Occasionally   O Frequently

5   Fewer situations trigger negative feelings like anger and jealousy.
    O Never   O Occasionally   O Frequently

6   Nervous habits like biting my nails or emotional eating are less or gone.
    O Never   O Occasionally   O Frequently

7   If I feel like crying or laughing, I let it out.
    O Never   O Occasionally   O Frequently

8   There's less chatter going on in my brain.
    O Never   O Occasionally   O Frequently

9   I'm recalling new memories of my childhood.
    O Never   O Occasionally   O Frequently

10 In general, I choose to be happy.
    O Never   O Occasionally   O Frequently

SCORING

Give yourself 5 points for every A answer, 3 points for every S, and 0 for each N; total your scores for the three sections. Pay special attention to the section that garnered your highest and lowest scores.

100 AND 150 POINTS: You're a 7–Day Yoga–Body Cleanse super sensational success! There's a good chance you followed the Cleanse with devotion and commitment and you're reaping its benefits. You don't need me to tell you how much your life has changed, and all for the best. So just read through this chapter and choose those exercises and treatments that you believe will help you feel even more awesome — *as if that's possible!* You'll be able to hold onto your groovy feeling longer if you change your diet permanently. Check through the recipes and try a few new dishes. If you say *adios* to sugar and processed foods forever and continue to care for your inner life, you'll be golden.

BETWEEN 100 AND 145 POINTS: Sure, you're feeling like a million bucks, but what if you could amp up your energy and boost your mood even more? Go over your quiz results and zoom in on the section(s) where you scored the lowest. If it's your spirit or your emotions, you can find the tools to fine-tune them in this chapter. You might need a bit more pampering or a more dedicated yoga practice or a concentrated daily meditation routine. Check it out and trust your intuition to lead you in the right direction. If your low score was in the body section, find an exercise routine that sparks your enthusiasm. Vow to stay away from toxic eating habits. If you have the desire and willpower, you might consider eliminating caffeine and alcohol permanently. I know that's asking a lot. Check out the post-cleanse menu choices and see what whets your appetite.

LESS THAN 100 POINTS: Hey, don't get down on yourself. Give yourself the cred you totally deserve for seeing the Cleanse to the end. You've come a long way, but you can travel an even greater distance to a healthier and happier place by using this chapter as a guide to the second phase of your cleanse. See if you're up for the challenge. If you're feeling super resistant, then I suggest you just concentrate on pampering treatments, meditation, and simple yoga poses. When your spirit is more fully renewed, you'll be psyched to detox even more. As a general rule, try to eat less, rest more, and boost your appreciation for who you are and how far you've come! I guarantee you're a "whole" lot better in every way. As a general rule, ease into eating. Check out the recipes in this chapter as a way to expand your repertoire of healthy fare. And most importantly, keep in mind these words of iconic comedienne Lucille Ball:

"You really have to love yourself to get anything done in this world."

Diet

Ending the Cleanse can be as profound an experience as maintaining it. Here are the general rules for making a smooth-as-soy transition:

- Break the Cleanse with easy-to-digest foods such as steamed or puréed vegetables or lightly sautéed greens, as well as proteins such as unsalted raw nuts, legumes, and eggs.

- Introduce regular foods back into your diet slowly.

- Continue to eat consciously: take your time preparing your meals, chewing your food, and being grateful for the abundance.

- Keep your portions a reasonable size and remember to use your cupped palm as an approximate measurement.

- Keep soups and juices as daily menu options.

- If you're planning on eating meat again, start with organic poultry rather than red meat.

- Opt for organic ingredients whenever possible.

Post-Cleanse Recipes

Here are some of my favorite recipes to ease you out of the Cleanse. That said, as long as you follow the general rules for post–detox, you can eat whatever makes your mouth water.

Breakfast

MORNING MILLET
MAKES: About 3 ½ cups

1¾ cups water

1 cup millet, rinsed and drained

¼ cup almond or soy milk

Maple syrup, to taste

1 teaspoon nuts of choice

1 teaspoon raisins

Bring the water to boil in a small pan over high heat. Toast the millet in a dry saucepan over medium heat until beige colored, and then add to the water. Reduce the heat to low and simmer until the water is completely absorbed. Stir occasionally. Remove from the heat and let stand for about 10 minutes. Put one serving (an open palm's worth) in your bowl and add soy or almond milk, maple syrup, and nuts and raisins. Enjoy! Share leftovers with friends or store the remaining millet in a tight-lidded container in refrigerator and reheat later.

QUINOA CEREAL
MAKES: 3 cups

Palm-sized serving of quinoa

Ground cinnamon

Honey or maple syrup

Fresh fruit

Prepare portion of quinoa, sprinkle with cinnamon, drizzle with honey or maple syrup, and add fresh fruit.

BOWL OF FRESH FRUIT – YOUR CHOICE!

GRANNY SMITH APPLE TOPPED WITH A TEASPOON OF ALMOND BUTTER

YUMMY MUFFINS FOR THE WEEK
MAKES: About 8 muffins

Olive oil, for greasing the muffin tin

1 cup rolled oats

1 cup oat flour

1 cup organic unsweetened applesauce

¼ cup chopped walnuts

¼ cup flaxseed meal

¼ cup organic honey

½ teaspoon shredded fresh ginger

Preheat the oven to 350°F. Lightly rub 8 cups of a 12-cup muffin tin with olive oil and set aside. Combine all the ingredients in a large bowl and stir well to combine. Scoop out mixture into the muffin tin cups, allowing about ⅓ cup for each muffin. Bake 20 minutes, or until the muffin tops are lightly browned. Serve warm.

STAY-CLEANSED OMELET
SERVES: 1 or 2

1 tablespoon plus 1 teaspoon olive oil

½ Vidalia onion, chopped

1 cup fresh organic spinach

2 organic free-range egg yolks

2 tablespoons water

Pinch of cayenne pepper

3 cloves garlic

1 avocado, sliced

Warm 1 tablespoon of the olive oil over medium heat and sauté the onions for 4 minutes; add the spinach and sauté until soft. Remove the vegetables to a small bowl. In a second small bowl, whisk the egg yolks, water, and cayenne. Add the remaining 1 teaspoon olive oil to the pan over medium heat. Add the egg mixture, and when the eggs start to firm up, add the vegetables to the middle of the omelet. Just before folding in half and serving, add the avocado.

Lunch

CHILLY CUCUMBER SOUP
SERVES: 1

2 cups peeled, chopped cucumber

2 tablespoons chopped chives or scallions

1 teaspoon chopped fresh dill

2 tablespoon extra-virgin olive oil

2 tablespoons water

sea salt and black pepper, to taste

Puree all the ingredients together in a blender until smooth.

HOT & CREAMY BROCCOLI SOUP
SERVES: 2

1 head broccoli, chopped

1 cup raw cashews, soaked in water for 1 hour

¼ teaspoon ground nutmeg

1 clove garlic

1 teaspoon freshly squeezed lemon

1 tablespoon extra-virgin olive oil

½ teaspoon dried thyme

sea salt and pepper, to taste

Bring about 1 inch of water to a boil in a saucepan and add the broccoli. Cook for 5 minutes, or until the broccoli is soft enough to be pierced by a fork. Drain the soaked cashews and place in a blender. Add the nutmeg, salt and pepper, garlic, lemon juice, and olive oil. Blend on high until smooth. Add the broccoli and pulse until it's chunky. Pour the mixture into a saucepan and add the thyme. Simmer for 5 minutes over medium heat and stir frequently. Serve.

AVOCADO & FENNEL SALAD
SERVES: 2

10 ounces organic arugula

4 to 5 kale leaves, de-stemmed and torn into pieces

½ cup torn basil leaves

1 bulb fennel, sliced thinly

1 avocado, sliced thinly

¼ cup plus 1 tablespoon extra-virgin olive oil

3 tablespoons apple cider vinegar

Juice of 1 lemon

Combine the arugula, kale, and basil in a large bowl. Drizzle over 1 tablespoon of the olive oil and mix the greens together with your hands until evenly coated. Toss in the fennel and avocado. In a separate bowl, mix the remaining ¼ cup olive oil, and the cider vinegar and lemon juice. Pour the dressing over the salad.

YUMMY YOGURT
SERVES: 1

Fresh fruit

1 tablespoon walnuts

1 (8-ounce) container plain whole-milk Greek yogurt

Add fresh fruit and nuts to the yogurt for intestine cleansing treat.

SPELT BREAD AND ALMOND BUTTER

MAKES: 2 large loaves

8 cups spelt flour

½ cup sesame seeds

½ teaspoon salt, or to taste

1 tablespoon blackstrap molasses

2 teaspoon baking soda

4¼ cups milk

Almond butter, to serve

Preheat the oven to 350°F. Grease two 9 x 5-inch loaf pans with olive oil or ghee. In a large bowl, mix together the spelt flour, sesame seeds, salt, molasses, baking soda, and milk until blended. Divide the batter between the two pans. Bake 1 hour and 10 minutes, or until golden brown. Cool for 30 minutes. To serve, spread almond butter on sliced bread. Freeze the second loaf. Newly baked spelt bread will stay fresh for 7 to 10 days. Do not refrigerate.

Snacks

BANANA-BLUEBERRY SMOOTHIE
SERVES: 1

1 cup fresh blueberries

½ apple, cored and chopped

1 ripe banana

½ teaspoon organic vanilla extract

Combine all ingredients in a blender and blend until smooth.

PINEAPPLE-BLUE SMOOTHIE
SERVES: 2

1 cup fresh or frozen organic blueberries

1 cup fresh or frozen organic pineapple chunks

1½ cups soy, rice, or whole cow's milk

Combine all ingredients in a blender and blend until smooth.

COOKED APPLES WITH CINNAMON
SERVES: 1

1 whole apple, cored and peeled

½ cup milk or soy or almond milk

5 teaspoons ground cinnamon

Handful nuts and seeds of choice

Dice the apple into small pieces. Combine the apples and milk in a sauté pan over low heat to cook. Add the cinnamon, nuts, and seeds. When the nuts and seeds brown, remove from the heat and serve warm.

HOTSY TOTSY EDAMAME HUMUS
SERVES: 2

3½ cups purified water, divided

1½ teaspoons sea salt, divided

1 cup frozen shelled edamame

½ cup sesame tahini

3 tablespoons extra-virgin olive oil

3 tablespoons fresh lemon juice

2 cloves garlic

½ teaspoon chili powder

Pinch cayenne pepper

Organic finger-sized carrots,
for dipping

Place 3 cups of the water and 1 teaspoon of the salt and bring to a boil. Add the edamame and bring back to a boil. Cook, uncovered, for a full 5 minutes. Drain and place in blender at high speed with all the remaining ingredients, including the remaining ½ cup water and ½ teaspoon salt, except the carrots. Put in small bowl. Dip carrots in the hummus.

GUACAMOLE
SERVES: 4 to 6

3 Hass avocados, finely chopped

4 ripe, juicy organic tomatoes, diced

½ teaspoon minced garlic

Bunch of cilantro, chopped

Juice of 1 lime

Sea salt, to taste

Gently mash the ingredients together. Dip flaxseed crackers or finger-sized carrots into the guacamole.

HOMEMADE GRANOLA BARS
MAKES: 10 bars

1 cup sunflower seeds

½ cup sesame seeds or hemp seeds

1 tablespoon flaxseeds

1½ tablespoons extra-virgin olive oil

2 tablespoons pure maple syrup or raw honey

1½ teaspoons ground cinnamon

2 tablespoons chopped dried fruit, like raisins or dried cranberries

Preheat the oven to 375°F. Combine the sunflower, hemp, and flaxseeds and stir together. Add the oil and maple syrup or honey, and blend again. Pour out into a bowl and add in the cinnamon and dried fruit. Work them in with your hands. Press the dough into a rimmed baking sheet. Bake for 15 to 20 minutes, until the tops are firm and lightly golden. Let cool until firm and cut into bars.

BUGS ON A LOG
Organic celery spread with almond butter or tahini and sprinkled with raisins.

Dinner

BANGIN' BORSCHT
SERVES: 2

3 tablespoons extra-virgin olive oil

3 small Vidalia onions, chopped

3 cloves garlic, minced

3 beets, shredded

3 carrots, shredded

8 cups purified water

1 tablespoon vegetable bouillon

Sea salt, to taste

Juice of ½ lemon

2 bay leaves

Handful of fresh parsley, chopped, plus more for garnish

Dollop of plain yogurt, for garnish

Warm the oil in a big soup pot over medium-high heat. Add the onions and garlic and sauté until translucent. Add the beets and carrots, followed by the water, vegetable bullion, salt, lemon juice, bay leaves, and a handful of chopped parsley. Bring to a boil over high heat, then reduce the heat to medium and cook for 1 hour. Serves four. Add a dollop of plain yogurt to each bowl and garnish with parsley. Refrigerate remainder before yogurt or garnish.

SUPERHEALTHY COBB SALAD

SERVES: 2 or 3

2 teaspoons extra-virgin olive oil

2 boneless, skinless organic free-range chicken breast halves *(optional)*

2 plum tomatoes, cut into wedges

½ yellow onion, sliced

1 ear corn

1 avocado, diced

2 hard-boiled egg whites, chopped

¼ cup crumbled goat cheese

8 cups torn lettuce leaves

DRESSING:

3 tablespoons nonfat Greek yogurt

¼ cup light buttermilk

½ teaspoon Dijon mustard

2 teaspoons fresh lemon juice

Pinch of sea salt and pepper

Preheat a grill to medium heat. To make the dressing, in a small bowl, whisk together the yogurt, buttermilk, Dijon, lemon juice, and salt and pepper. Set aside. To prepare the caramelized onion, the oil in a small skillet over low heat and add the sliced onion. Cook on low for about 20 minutes, or until the onions are golden and caramelized. Remove from the heat and set aside. Grill the chicken breast until cooked through, 15 to 18 minutes. While the chicken is cooking, add the corn and tomatoes to the grill, and grill until the chicken is cooked through. Once chicken is done, remove everything from the grill. Slice the chicken and remove the corn from the cob. In large shallow bowls or on roomy dinner plates, arrange the lettuce, chicken, tomatoes, corn, onions, avocado, egg whites, and goat cheese. Drizzle the dressing over the top.

CLASSIC COD AND SPINACH
SERVES: 4

1 tablespoon ghee

3 tablespoons pine nuts

3 tablespoons fresh lemon juice, divided

4 (5-ounce) cod fillets

½ teaspoon sea salt

¼ teaspoon freshly ground black pepper

3 teaspoons extra-virgin olive oil, divided

2 minced garlic cloves

2 bunches fresh organic spinach, washed and trimmed

lemon wedges

Melt the ghee in large, heavy nonstick skillet over medium heat. Add the pine nuts and 2 tablespoons of the lemon juice, and stir; cook 1 minute or until the nuts are golden brown. Remove from the pan and set aside. Season the fish with salt and pepper. Add 2 teaspoons of the oil to the skillet over medium-high heat. Add the fish; cook 2 minutes per side, until it flakes. Transfer to a platter and place the nuts on top of the fish. Tent with foil to keep warm. Wipe the skillet clean with a paper towel. Warm the remaining 1 teaspoon oil over medium heat. Add the garlic and spinach; cook 5 minutes, stirring until the spinach wilts. Add the remaining 1 tablespoon lemon juice; cook 1 minute to blend the flavors. Place the spinach on a serving platter and top with the fish. Serve with lemon wedges.

TASTY TANDOORI CHICKEN
SERVES: 4

1½ cups plain reduced-fat Greek yogurt

2 tablespoon grated onion

1 tablespoon grated peeled fresh ginger

1 tablespoon canola oil

1 teaspoon ground cumin

½ teaspoon cayenne pepper

¼ teaspoon ground turmeric

3 garlic cloves, minced

4 (6-ounce) skinless, boneless organic, free-range chicken breast halves

½ teaspoon sea salt

ghee

Combine the first 8 ingredients in a heavy-duty zip-top plastic bag. Add the chicken to the bag and seal. Marinate in the refrigerator 2 hours, turning occasionally. Place a small roasting pan in oven. Preheat the broiler to high. Remove the chicken from the bag; discard the marinade. Sprinkle both sides of the chicken evenly with salt. Coat the preheated pan with ghee and add the chicken. Broil in the lower third of the oven for 15 minutes or until done, turning after 7 minutes.

Desserts

THE TURTLE BLUES
MAKES: 5

7 tablespoons (2.5 ounces) 60% cocoa bittersweet organic chocolate chips or carob chips

¼ cup wild blueberries *(sold in produce section)*

¼ cup sliced almonds

Melt the chocolate or carob chips. Stir in the blueberries and nuts, then drop In 5 rounded tablespoons onto parchment paper. Refrigerate for 2 to 4 minutes or until firm.

MINT POMEGRANATE PARFAIT
SERVES: 1

2 teaspoons thinly sliced fresh mint

½ cup nonfat Greek yogurt

⅓ cup pomegranate arils *(the juicy covering over the seed)*

Fold the mint into the yogurt. Layer the yogurt mixture and pomegranate arils in a clear dessert dish.

HONEY FRUIT CUP
SERVES: 1

1 cup fresh fruit *(such as pineapple, kiwi, and assorted berries)*

1 small lime

½ tablespoon honey

Place the fruit in a medium serving bowl. Zest and juice the lime. In a small bowl, whisk ½ teaspoon lime zest and ½ tablespoon lime juice into the honey until well blended; drizzle over the fruit salad and toss gently to mix.

Follow Up with At-Home Treatments

Did any treatments make your heart sing and your soul soar? Well, splurge and book another one. If it was a homemade pampering treatment, why not make it a habit? Remember, you deserve to feel THIS good.

Beautifiers

Instant Shiatsu Face-Lift

Put your fingers near the center of your cheeks at the place where the bone protrudes, and move them down slightly, then slightly out toward your ears. Stimulating these points can increase circulation and relax the drawn or fatigued areas around your mouth and eyes, soothing fatigued eyes and reducing puffiness.

Sun Spot Remover

If you have visible sun damage like spots or freckles, you might want to try dabbing the area daily with fresh lemon juice which acts as a bleach. Some people find the lemon too acidic and have irritating reactions. If this is the case for you, of course, discontinue use. Always follow with a natural moisturizer.

Lip Healer

If your lips get chapped, you can find relief by making your own balm. Simply melt a dollop of beeswax in a double boiler with 3 teaspoons of almond oil. Stir well, cook, cool and apply to your lips. This balm can be safely stored in a tight container for a day or two. For natural lip color, mash berries with a bit of aloe vera. Commercial lipstick, when used regularly can drain the lips of their natural colors.

Sensible Cellulite Treatment

Cellulite is plain old fat that has bunched up in little pockets. The popular procedure of vacuuming appeals more to vanity than good health. Whether or not this mechanical shortcut holds lasting results is still open to debate. But if you are really serious about shedding cellulite, eat plenty of fresh fruits and vegetables, which detoxify the body, and drink lots of water. Water tends to open up the blood vessels just below the skin level where most cellulite hides and helps flush it out. At the same time, reduce the salt in your diet. Salt makes your body retain water and adds to the cellulite condition. Some light muscle-building workouts tone up the tissues where cellulite ordinarily collects, so it doesn't have room to form, meanwhile, reinforce exercise by dry bushing your skin with rosemary, sandalwood, juniper, or lemon oil dabbed on a brush. Any one of these essences will penetrate the skin and work to improve circulation and detoxify. Although it's good to massage cellulite-prone areas like the butt and thighs, go easy on the skin. Cellulite-dappled spots are usually very tender. Brush gently until pink, take a bath with one of the detox formulas and then massage the cellulite area again.

Wrinkle Remedies

Red wine is an ancient Roman remedy for wrinkled skin; the wine contains a natural acid that smoothes superficial lines. Mix 1 tablespoon of red wine with 2 tablespoons of honey. Smooth it onto your face, and allow it to dry; then rinse. Be sure to follow up with a moisturizer with anti-aging emollients like jojoba, cocoa butter, olive oil, or aloe vera oil.

OR

Mix ½ cup of mashed pineapple with 1 tablespoon of honey, and apply the mixture to your face. Relax for 10 minutes and then wash with cool water.

OR

Brewer's yeast is also touted as effective in smoothing skin and minimizing laugh lines. Make a paste with brewer's yeast and olive oil. Allow it to dry completely before rinsing off your face.

Yogurt Cooling Mask

Mix 3 teaspoons of plain organic yogurt and 3 tablespoons of honey, which locks in moisture. Smooth onto your clean skin and leave on for 15 minutes. Remove with cool spring water. Now apply pure aloe vera juice with a cotton ball. Aloe vera not only cleanses your skin but also heals and detoxifies it.

Superconditioning Hair Pack

Mix together ½ cup of mayonnaise, ½ of a mashed ripe avocado, and two teaspoons of lemon juice. Rinse your hair with warm water; then apply the hair pack. Cover your hair with a plastic bag (or an old shower cap) and leave on for 15 minutes. Shampoo out with your favorite organic product.

Aromatic Hair Shiner

In a small pot, heat ¼ cup of almond oil until it's comfortably warm. Mix in 5 drops each of chamomile, lavender, and patchouli essential oils. Once the mixture has cooled to a comfortable temperature, apply it to your damp hair. After 15 minutes, shampoo until you get a good, vigorous lather going, then rinse.

Body & Soul

Self-Massage

This requires the proper setting. Warmth, comfort, quiet, and low light are all essential. Find a position that is relaxing and comfortable. Lying on your back or side may be good for some parts, but of others it's easier to sit or kneel down. Have a fragrant body lotion or massage oil ready for use when you need it. Work slowly and rhythmically, closing your eyes so that you can focus all your attention on sensation. You need have no set routine, but I found the following technique to be the most soothing and enlightening.

- ❦ Begin by exploring your face thoroughly, as if you were a blind person learning to recognize it for the first time. Work more deeply with your thumbs and fingers around any areas of tension, like the jaw muscles or eye sockets.

- ❦ Repeatedly comb your fingers through your hair, or gently rub your scalp, as if you were shampooing. Place your hands on top of your head, fingers spread apart. Press down, and rub your scalp in a small, circular motion. Move your fingers a half-inch closer to your forehead and repeat. Continue massaging until you reach your hairline; place the index fingers on the temples and massage the area. This massage is immensely relaxing and totally effective for relieving toxic tension, especially if you're the kind of person (like me) who tends to live in her head.

❧ If you spend a lot of time in front of a computer, your shoulders and neck are probably tight and knotted. Massage both shoulders at once, or do first one side with your opposite hand, then the other side. Starting at the base of your neck, massage along your shoulder until you reach the top of your arm. Press fingertips deeply into the back of your shoulder as you massage.

❧ Exploring one of your own hands with the other is an unusual sensation at first, since we're used to shaking or holding hands with others. But it gives us the unique opportunity to see how it feels to give and receive at the same time. Try working your thumb into the fleshy areas of the palm and stretching each finger.

❧ We also often neglect our feet, forgetting the service our peds do every day. Yet massaging your own feet can be immensely beneficial and relaxing. Try working across the sole with your fingers or thumb or stretching and pulling your toes.

❧ Complete your massage by lying down and totally relaxing for 20 minutes.

Power of Prayer

For many, spiritual healing conjures up images of suspect media evangelists. But that perception may be fading as the effectiveness of prayer gains a measure of scientific respectability. Over a decade ago, the National Institutes of Health gave a big-bucks grant to a researcher to study the role of prayer in curing drug and alcohol addiction. Not surprisingly, dozens of other studies followed.

In fact, in his landmark book *Healing Words*, Dr. Larry Dossey, who gave up his practice as an internist to write about spirituality and healing, reviewed more than 130 studies on prayer. He found that the research showed prayer positively affected high blood pressure, asthma, heart attacks, headaches, and anxiety. According to the studies, people who pray for themselves and others achieve effects that are scientifically provable. Dossey added that it's not necessary to be religious or to believe in God, Goddess, Allah, Krishna, Brahma, the Tao, the Universal Mind, or the Almighty for prayer to work. One must instead put their faith in the power of prayer.

How does prayer relate to detoxing? Well, you can ask for the strength to change, grow, cleanse, and be in control of your life. Or, you might pray to share your growth with others, to let you love those who support your endeavor, as well as those who may try to put obstacles in your way. You might pray to fill your heart with forgiveness for your past indulgences, and encourage your spirit to continue to work towards purification. *Amen.*

Working the Koan: How to Be Your Own Buddha

A koan is an ancient saying or story that a Zen Buddhist teacher offers. Surprisingly, what the student answers is of little consequence. What's more important is the journey. The koan is meant to bring the mind into deepening awareness. Indeed, practicing these meditations will help focus your mind.

Here's a classic to consider:
"What is the sound of one hand clapping?"

Sit with this question in meditation. When you think you have the answer, think again.

Post-Cleanse Yoga

As you know by now, your circulatory, digestive, and lymphatic systems help your body rid itself of toxins. Yoga poses can bump up their effectiveness, especially after a cleanse. Here's my favorite to do after the intensive week has ended:

Supine Spinal Twist Pose (Supta Matsyendrasana): Lie on your back and bend your knees while keeping the soles of your feet firmly planted on the floor. Now lift your hips slightly off the floor and shift them about an inch to your right. Draw your right knee into your chest and extend the left leg on the floor. Drop your right knee over to the left side of your body. Next, open your right arm to the right side in line with your shoulder. Rest your left hand on your right knee; then turn your head to the right, bringing your gaze over the right shoulder. You can work on releasing your left knee and your right shoulder to the floor. Hold 5 to 10 breaths before drawing your right knee back into your chest and repeating on the other side.

Journal Reflections

After the Yoga-Body Cleanse it's likely that you're in a state of heightened perception and may be experiencing greater clarity. Try not to let this supersensitive time slip by. It could be your chance to work through major breakthroughs on issues in your life that have been holding you back. Take time to sit in silence with a pen and journal. Allow your mind to open and bring your heart along for the ride. Post-cleanse is also an ideal time to write down your intentions for the future.

The quieter you become, the more you can hear.   —Ram Dass

CHAPTER SIX

WEEKEND WARRIOR

At times it was really hard for me to stick to the week-long Cleanse, but I managed and was over-the-top thrilled for mustering the discipline. It was so worth it. For the next three months, I pretty much felt awesome. I tried some of the post-cleanse recipes, was able to reduce my sugar and alcohol intake, eliminated caffeine, put a mini-meditation and yoga practice into my daily routine, rose with the sun, and felt generally uplifted. Of course, I still noticed if things didn't go my way, but those old destructive feelings of self-blame and disappointment didn't stick. Instead I sort of let it just flow. I even had a couple of mind-blowing "ah hah" moments. Also, lots of people remarked about how great I looked, probably because I maintained a 7-pound weight loss.

But now, well, I'm starting to slack off. I find excuses for why I really need that morning cup of coffee. I'm feeling more of those familiar prickles of anxiety and anger, and my inner dialogue is whispering, "You don't have time to meditate or do yoga." So, I skip it. Worst of all is the undeniable fact that

I've lost my energy. I'm feeling run down and lethargic. On top of it, when I look in the mirror the face staring back at me looks lackluster. What happened to my glow?

Is this you?

Well, nothing lasts forever, right? Some folks do manage to sustain the same daily routine they used during their detox cleanse. But that's their nature. They have the kind of internal discipline that can withstand all kinds of outside pressures and temptations. Most of us don't have wills made of iron, so why get down on yourself? Besides, guilt won't get you anywhere. But a 24-hour Weekend Warrior Cleanse (which is more of a fast than a detox diet) will!

This quick detoxification trip will give you back many of the same benefits as the longer cleanse. Even better, it can expel poisons from your body without those annoying hunger pangs. The short cleanse/fast is especially beneficial if you've fallen back into old destructive patterns of consuming alcohol, smoking, overeating, or stressing out.

Science Says Fasting Can Be Fabulous

There's been a lot of research on fasting recently, and studies point to some major health benefits including reducing the risk of cancer, cardiovascular diseases, diabetes, immune disorders, as well as slowing down the process of aging. Other health benefits include stress resistance and an increased life span, not to mention weight loss. On the down side, some studies reported testiness by the subjects while fasting. But you needn't worry about getting short-tempered, since the Weekend Warrior semifast is short and sweet, and centers on your heart not in your stomach.

Buddhist monks and nuns following the Vinaya rules commonly don't eat after their noon meal. This isn't considered a fast but rather a disciplined regimen aiding in meditation and good health.

Preparation

If you've decided to become a Weekend Warrior, you need to prepare for it at the beginning of the week, on Monday. If you jump rather than ease into it slowly, you might end up getting nauseous, headachy, and exhausted.

Here's what you'll need to eat less of, or even better, eliminate, prior to becoming a Weekend Warrior:

- Sugar
- Caffeine
- Alcohol
- Processed foods
- Meat, chicken, fish
- Dairy

Here's what you can bump up:

- ✤ Water
- ✤ Greens
- ✤ Meditation/Yoga
- ✤ Pampering
- ✤ Rest

● ●

WATCH OUT FOR THIS COMPLICATION!

Changes in blood chemistry during fasting in combination with certain medications may have dangerous effects, such as increased chance of acetaminophen poisoning! If you're on *any* meds, speak with your doctor before fasting even one single day.

● ●

Think Ahead

Mark your Warrior Weekend on your calendar well in advance. I recommend beginning the fast-cleanse on Friday night and breaking it on Sunday. During the pre-Cleanse weekdays you should have nothing to do other than taming your life. Disco dancing at the hottest club in town is definitely out. So is a meal of sushi and sake or a fast food burger deluxe (or even a meatball)! Now is not the time to break up with your boyfriend or spend the weekend with your extended family. And for heaven's sake, don't schedule any physical challenges such as starting a new spin class. In other words, don't engage in any activity that challenges you physically or emotionally.

Boosting the Warrior Spirit

To help prepare, try dishes from these sample menus two or three days before your Warrior Cleanse to allow your digestive system to relax into a state of semifast. You can choose one or more dishes for each meal (recipes are in Chapter Four). Whatever you choose to eat, don't stuff yourself thinking you'll be fasting in only a few days. Keep the palm-portion rule in mind and, in general, dine lightly.

Breakfast

Skip morning coffee or tea and instead opt for hot water with lemon. If you're a heavy caffeine drinker, limit to one cup daily, then reduce to half a cup, and finally eliminate completely.

Choose from the following meals:

- Any combination of banana and berry smoothies
- Fruit cup
- Steel-cut oatmeal with seeds and nuts
- Whole-grain toast with peanut or almond butter
- Sprouted-grain cereal with soy milk

Morning Snack

Choose from the following options:

- Fruit smoothie
- Homemade popcorn with sea salt
- Seaweed snacks
- Handful of nuts and seeds

Lunch

Choose from the following options:

- Whole-grain crackers and guacamole
- Humus and carrots or whole-grain crackers
- Green salad (add nuts or grains to taste) dressed with spritz of fresh lemon
- A light vegetable broccoli, spinach, or split pea soup made without dairy

Afternoon Snack

Choose from the following options:

- Smoothie
- Protein nut bar (as long as it's made without sugar)

Dinner

Choose from the following options:

- Roasted Beets (page 100)
- Green salad (add nuts or grains to taste) dressed with spritz of fresh lemon
- Sautéed green vegetables (mixed or a single vegetable)
- Vegetable soup
- Guacamole (page 134)
- Cooked vegetables and quinoa
- Soup and sprouted bread

Dessert

Choose from the following options:

- Fruit in season
- Cup of herb tea
- Remember to drink lots of purified water!

Weekend Warrior Fast Begins

Friday Evening

Eat a light dinner and finish by 7 p.m.

You may sip a cup of herb tea before bed, but otherwise just drink purified water until sleep.

Spend your evening quietly and, if possible, in solitude. Turn off all electronics.

Feng Shui Your Space

You don't need to devote an entire room for meditation. Dedicate a space in the corner of your bedroom, office, or living room. Since I live in an open loft space, I sit in my laundry room because it's the only room with a door. The most important aspect of a meditation area is that it's a sanctuary where you can relax your mind and connect with your inner being through meditation, prayer, contemplation, and yoga, or write in your journal. By employing the ancient art of feng shui, you can design the area to create a positive flow. Represent the four elements: earth, air, fire, and water. A plant represents the earth element. Air is often represented by burning incense. Candles represent fire. Water can be represented by a small bowl of water. Most importantly, create a comfortable place where you can sit or lie down. You may prefer a simple mat, one or two floor cushions, a low stool, or a straight-backed chair. Whichever works best for you. It's a personal choice.

Keep Your Heart Open

What better place to look for self-awareness and strength than at your heart center? This yoga pose helps to free your heart and open new channels of understanding, energy and love—the perfect trifecta for the Weekend Warrior Cleanse.

Yoga Supported Bridge Pose (Setu Bandha Sarvangasana)

Have a block or blanket(s) near your mat. Lie on your back. Bend your knees, bringing them close enough to your butt so that you can touch them with your fingertips. With your arms along your sides and palms pressing into the mat, roll up one vertebra at time. Position your support under your back. As a variation, try using a block first on the flat side. Roll down, and return to bridge supporting your back with the block at medium height. Roll down one vertebra at time and, if you have no back problems, roll up into bridge a third time, using the block at its full height. Hold each pose for 30 seconds to 1 minute or more. Release one vertebra at a time to the mat and lie supine.

Meditation

Set a timer for the period you want to sit. Mine is routinely set at 30 minutes. Decide whether you'll be sitting on a cushion or chair. Settle in with a straight back and then quiet down and watch your breath. Feel it on the tip of your nostril. In and out. In and out. Allow your thoughts to come and go. Just watch. Just breathe. Now envision your heart in the center of your chest and simply be present to whatever you experience. Visualize your heart expanding and getting brighter with a white light. Allow it to extend outside your chest. Allow the energy to connect above, around and beyond you. As your heart opens, thoughts may come and go … that's okay. Welcome all … and then let it go.

Muslce-Relaxing Bath

Hang a "Do Not Disturb" sign on your bathroom door. Place beeswax candles strategically around the tub so their lights flicker reflectively on the water. Add a few drops of lavender oil to the bath. Keep the bathwater on a slow trickle to maintain the temperature. While in the tub, close your eyes and imagine drifting on a lake or river. Envision your heart ascending skyward. When you're finished bathing, don't hurry out of the water. After your soak, turn on the shower and stay there, resting your head on your knees for a few minutes. Come back into the world.

HINT: *Before your bath, change the sheets on your bed. After bathing, lie in bed luxuriously naked.*

Journal

Even if you haven't written in your journal since you ended your original cleanse, now is a good time to bring it out again and write down your thoughts. The only rule is to avoid self-critical words. You don't need to lecture or blame yourself. Opt for expressions of encouragement. Write down your own affirmations or contemplate these special fasting affirmations:

> *Every hour that I fast I become happier, healthier and have more energy.*

> *Hour by hour, my body is cleansing and purifying itself.*

When I fast I am using the same method for physical, mental and spiritual purification that the greatest spiritual leaders have used throughout the ages.

Go to sleep early, before 10 p.m., and *dream on!*

Saturday

Today you're in full-blast Weekend Warrior mode. Remind yourself that as a Warrior you've *chosen* to release toxins and heal your body. You'll be going deeper inside your psyche, removing emotional armor but strengthening your commitment and discipline. Hopefully, without judgment, you'll also be able to examine your motives and reactions to whatever arises. Don't be surprised if a revelation surges forth. Open your heart and welcome change.

Your time is your own. You can choose suggested activities whenever the spirit touches you. You may decide to do nothing more than sit quietly or go for a long walk. Just remember to stay present and engage with your senses. No matter what's happening, where you're going or what you're doing, try to stay in the here and now.

Morning

1   Rise with the sun.

2   Recall any dreams and write them in your journal.

3 Remind yourself today you will not be eating any solid foods. With an open heart, you'll be releasing the old and welcoming in the new.

4 Scrape your tongue.

5 Enjoy a cup of hot water with a squeeze of fresh lemon.

6 Stretch with yoga.

Yoga Triangle Pose (Trikonasana)

This pose stretches the muscles of the inner thighs and back, opening your heart across your chest. Assume a wide-legged stance, with your toes pointed forward. Turn your left foot so that the heel points toward the arch of your right foot. On an inhale, lift your arms parallel to the floor. On an exhale, bend forward over the left leg. Drop the left hand down the leg, all the way to the floor if possible. Turn your head to look up at the other hand. Keep your spine straight. Hold the pose for five to ten breaths; then repeat on the other side.

Enjoy a big glass of purified water!

Return to Open Heart Meditation

Sit in an upright and seated posture, but be comfortable. Relax your tummy. Now center your on the flow of your breath. Keep your attention on your breath, but notice how your mind is calming down. Now focus on the heart space in the center of your chest. Bring your breath into it and then release your breath out of it. As this takes place, just notice how, at the same time, you can experience your heart gently opening and then softening. Every breath offers you more

… and more … release. You can add to the experience by whispering to yourself silently, "My heart is opening. My heart is softening. I can feel love." You may experience great joy or even a wave of deep sadness. Let the feelings come and go; just keep breathing into your heart space. Stay here. When you are ready, take a deep breath and let it go. Gently open your eyes. Try to take this open heart space throughout the day.

Morning Warrior Ultratoxin Release Shower and Scrub

Exfoliating gets rid of all the dead cells that hold toxins and leaves your skin soft and glowing. Before entering the shower, rub your body down with either room- temperature extra-virgin olive oil or flaxseed oil. Pay special attention to your elbows, knees, and heels. Now step carefully into a steamy shower. (Be careful not to slip!) Scrub your skin in a circular motion using a loofah or a scratchy bath scrubber, or a firm brush. After waiting for a few minutes, rinse off with warm water and pat dry with a soft towel. If your skin feels too oily, you can wash it off with some organic soap, but it's not necessary because skin usually absorbs all the oil; this process benefits your dry skin most. Your skin should now feel soft, moisturized, and creamy.

REMINDER: Drink plenty of purified water today. It's especially important to have a full glass of water after a toxin-release shower and scrub!

Afternoon

Any time in the afternoon, preferably around three o'clock, sip a glass of this green juice.

GREEN DREAM

1 head celery
1 teaspoon fresh ginger
1 green apple, cored

Chop the ingredients into small pieces that your juicer feed tube or blender will accept. Start with the celery. Pour into a glass and add enough purified water to make a 16 ounce serving. Drink up!

Enjoy a Nap

Are you feeling sleepy? Some people find their energy is percolating when they're Weekend Warriors and others feel waves of fatigue. Remember, no judgment. If you're in the latter camp, don't fight the feeling. Your body knows what it needs. Besides, napping doesn't just feel good—studies show it can also recharge your body and add fuel to your psyche. A study of 24,000 adults done by the Harvard School of Public Health found that nappers were 40 percent less likely to die of heart disease than those who don't regularly take naps. Even if napping is unusual for you, you'll still reap major benefits. Daytime napping for 45 minutes has been shown to lower blood pressure, according to 2011 research at Allegheny College.

It's best to start your nap sometime between noon and 1 p.m., or when you find your energy drooping. But avoid taking your naps too late in the day. After around 3 p.m., daytime sleep will start to interfere with night sleep. To enhance your nap, remind yourself to dream before dozing off. Try to recall any dreams immediately upon awakening. You might want to record them in your journal.

- -

PER CHANCE TO DREAM

A new study conducted at the Center for Sleep and Cognition at Beth Israel Deaconess Medical Center in Boston, Massachusetts, suggests that an afternoon power nap may boost your ability to process and store information *tenfold* — but only if you dream while you're asleep.

- -

Get Fresh Air

Of course it's more appealing to go outside when the weather is lovely, but you may not be cleansing on a stunning spring day. Don't let that stop you from going outdoors. You're a warrior! You can enjoy the natural elements no matter what they are. Fresh air provides you with a steady supply of oxygen, which is needed by your brain and every single cell of your body. If you stay indoors for a long period of time, you'll end up breathing in the same air over and over again.

Just be sure to dress appropriately for the weather. Wear sunscreen in the summer and light, all-natural fabrics that allow your skin to breathe if it's warm out. These include silk, cotton, or linen. Wear appropriately warm clothes in the winter. You might feel especially chilly while fasting, so put on extra layers. Consider taking a leisurely walk of at least 45 minutes. Notice your thoughts, then let them go. Practice not holding on to any mental loops. Try once again to be in the moment. Note what your senses are experiencing. Hey, did you bring along a bottle of water?

Praised by my Lord, for our sister water.

— St. Francis of Assisi (Canticle of the Sun)

Awakening the Senses

ALL HEARING: This means listening to the whole range and variety of sound vibrations that surround us. It's not just our playlist that can affect mood; every noise that enters our soul leaves its mark. If you train yourself to appreciate all sounds, you'll be less likely to regard noise as an irritation and be more likely to embrace it as a living experience.

Try this exercise: Sit comfortably near a window. Close your eyes and remain very still until you can hear the noise in your head. Now open up to include sounds in the room. Follow this by including the sounds in your ear and on the street, and finally more distant sounds.

ALL SEEING: Although we possess a wide field of vision, most of us focus on one small area at a time.

Try this exercise: Begin to pay attention to your outer, or peripheral, vision, which will lead you to a wider perspective.

Try to see without passing judgment. There is no "Oh, this is beautiful" or "This is unpleasant." There just is.

ALL TASTING: Here's an opportunity to drink another glass of water.

Sip it slowly, savoring the flavor of each drop in your mouth. Feel it against your tongue, your gums, the back of your throat; sense each drop as it slides down.

ALL SMELLING: Gather together strong-smelling natural objects like flowers, herbs, or organic soap (avoid fruit and other food that will perk up your appetite).

Close your eyes and pick up the objects one at a time. Allow yourself to absorb the aroma of each item.

ALL TOUCHING: Select some objects as different in weight and texture as you can find. The collection might include a shell, silk scarf, pumice stone, a piece of ice—you get the idea. Place what you've chosen on a tabletop. Close your eyes, pick up each item in turn, and explore it thoroughly, noticing any difference in textures and temperature.

Our sense of touch provides a vital source of information about our "state of being" and is a huge source of pleasure. By being attuned to the "feel" of the full experience rather than touching mechanically, our overall awareness in enriched.

Evening

Enjoy a hot cup of chamomile tea, preferably brewed from fresh leaves.

Be prepared to go to bed when the sun sets. If this is the winter, you might be tucking in by 7:30, and that's okay. When you're fasting, your body naturally wants to follow the rhythms of the day. In summer, of course, you'll be heading to bed later.

According to the National Sleep Foundation you can improve your sleep by designing an environment to establish the conditions you need for sleep: cool, quiet, dark, comfortable, and free of interruptions. Also check your room for noise or other distractions. Consider using blackout curtains, eye shades, ear plugs, and "white noise" makers like humidifiers, fans, and other devices. Make sure you're sleeping on bedding made of 100 percent natural fabrics. Keep your dream journal by the side of your bed in case you awaken recalling your nocturnal wanderings.

Acknowledge

Give yourself the credit you deserve, first for recognizing you needed to clean up your act again; second, for having the discipline and spirit to be a Weekend Warrior; and third for honoring your body and soul. Experience the gratitude you are feeling. Let it wash through you.

Sweet dreams!

Sunday

Congratulations Weekend Warrior! It's a new morning! A new day! And a new YOU!

Still, begin the day with your usual detox routine:

- 🌿 Rise with the sun.

- 🌿 Recall any dreams and write them in your journal.

- 🌿 Scrape your tongue.

- 🌿 Enjoy a cup of hot water with a squeeze of fresh lemon.

You can ease out of your fast in a similar way that you moved into it. Look at Friday's breakfast, lunch, dinner, and snack options, and choose from among them. No matter what you eat, you'll want to keep your portions small. Eat slowly, pay attention to each bite, and chew generously.

Review

Take Sunday slowly and deliberately. Be conscious of how your fast has affected you. If you've had any revelations, you may want to write them down in your journal. Avoid scheduling any taxing activities and, if possible, spend the day in solitude. You'll reap the most benefits if you give yourself another day to pamper your body and spirit, explore your senses, and generally revel in your life of renewal. Lucky you!

Yoga

Fish Pose (Matsyasana): This pose will help you open your heart to gratitude.

Lie on your back on top of a mat. Come up onto your elbows. Slide your body toward the back of the mat while keeping your forearms in place and puffing up your chest.

Drop the crown of your head back to the floor, opening your throat. If you're a beginner, place a blanket or block under your head if the crown does not comfortably come to the floor. To come out, press strongly into your forearms and raise your head off the floor. Release your upper body to the floor.

Naikan Meditation

This particular meditation practice was developed by Yoshimoto Ishin, a Japanese Buddhist monk. It means "inside looking" or "introspection" and is a structured method of self-reflection. If you were on a retreat it would be led by a trained counselor from dawn until night every day for a week. This is obviously a very abbreviated version to help keep your heart open and seal in gratitude after your Weekend Warrior Cleanse. Even in this short form, it can help you to examine your life in relationship to your immediate family and closest friends. For many, this isn't easy. That's exactly why it's so juicy and rewarding. Thanks to your fast, you're clear and strong enough to be able to do it.

While meditating, thank your mother with deep appreciation. Remember all she has done for you to the best of her ability. From there, move on to your father, siblings, lovers, and close friends. The rewards of a Naikan meditation can be immediate, helping you to nurture a deeply felt sense of gratitude and appreciation for your life and for all the gifts you receive daily. These gifts, you may realize, have always been here, but you may not have appreciated them before.

If the only prayer you said in your whole life was "thank you," that would suffice. — Meister Eckhart, 13th century mystic

The rest of your day should be spent in relaxation and reflection. The most important rule is to avoid stress if possible.

Clay Detox Bath

Close your day with this relaxing detoxing bath.

½ cup Epsom salt

3 tablespoons of lavender essential oil

½ cup bentonite clay *(bentonite forms from weathering of volcanic ash)*

Pour in the Epsom salts and essential oil as the water fills the tub. While this is happening, vigorously mix the clay into a small amount of water until the clumps are mostly dissolved. Do not use metal for this. Instead mix with a plastic or wooden spoon in a glass jar. Add the clay mix to the bath and soak for at least 20 minutes. Or mix the clay with a small amount of water to make a paste. Stand in the tub full of water and rub the clay mix all over your body to create a skin mask and let dry for 5 minutes before sitting down. This provides direct contact with the skin and effectively pulls toxins from the body. Soak in bath for at least 20 minutes, or as long as desired. While soaking, use a washcloth to scrub any remaining clay off the skin. This bath is great for removing any remainder of toxins as the clay binds to heavy metals and the Epsom salts help pull a variety of toxins from the body while replenishing magnesium levels.

Tuck in to bed when the sun sets.

If you're wondering *"How will I know when it's time to be a Weekend Warrior again?"*

You'll know.

CHAPTER SEVEN

KEEPING IT REAL

Life is a series of natural and spontaneous changes. Don't resist them — that only creates sorrow. Let reality be reality. Let things flow naturally forward in whatever way they like.

— Lao Tzu

Let's say you completed the 7 Day Yoga-Body Cleanse and a few months later you followed with the Weekend Warrior program. You appreciate how much better you feel and you're hoping to leap to another level. You want to experience your post-cleanse high 24/7! You want to feel like you're cooking with boundless energy *all* the time! You want to soar out of bed *every* morning and always face the day with joyous anticipation! You want to live in a toxin-free environment and do everything possible to make that happen! You want to eat only 100 percent natural, organic, unprocessed, unsweetened food and always consume it *slowly* and meditatively at every single meal! You want to remember your dreams in exquisite detail! You want to do yoga at least twice a day — no exceptions! You want to be *rid* of all those icky reactions like sadness, disappointment, jealousy, impatience, and anger *once and for all*!

Be Real: Tame Expectations

To keep expectations in perspective, consider what the Dali Lama, His Holiness of Happiness, told a reporter for *Time magazine* when asked about maintaining joy *all* the time:

Reporter: *Do you ever feel angry or outraged?*
His Holiness: *Oh, yes, of course. I'm a human being. Generally speaking, if a human being never shows anger, then I think something's wrong. He's not right in the brain.*

So, as long as we're human and "right in the brain," there will always be ups and downs. Life will present itself with challenges and sometimes we'll rise to them in our glory and sometimes we'll fall short of the mark. If your boyfriend dumps you or your boss has been on the war path and in turn, you devour a pint of ice cream, who can blame you? There will be times when we can adhere to healthy habits (including diet, exercise, meditation, and pampering) and other times when we'll feel overwhelmed by a particular issue and all those good intentions will go down the drain like so much dirty bath water.

If that's the case, and it is, how can we embrace our "messy" humanity, enjoy the rich, unpredictable juiciness of life—and then get back on a healthy routine sooner rather than later?

No judgment!
This perspective can change your life.

How to Tame Judgment

Begin by sharpening your awareness. Throughout the course of the day, note when you make judgments, when you have expectations, and when things don't live up to them. Over time, you'll notice this more and more, and be more conscious of these types of thoughts.

Take a deep breath each time you notice a judgment or expectation. Then tell yourself, "No expectations, no good or bad." Repeat this, breathing in, breathing out, letting go of the judgment or expectation.

Try to see things as they are. Be curious rather than reactive. Try to put yourself in other people's shoes rather than labeling them. Also, look at the landscape of your own life without the filter of judgments or expectations. It isn't "good" or "bad." It just is, in this moment.

Take what comes. Experience it. React appropriately, without overreacting because it isn't as you hoped or wanted. You can't control your life, or how others behave, but you can control how you react.

REMEMBER: Everything takes practice. No judgment.

Be Real: Acknowledge Pitfalls

While looking through the following Pitfall List you may recognize aspects of your life that are sabotaging the long-term benefits of your Yoga–Body Cleanse. Stay open and try to approach these possibilities without blaming yourself. Remember: No judgment!

CLUTTER: You're not enough of a packrat to star on the popular reality show Hoarders, but if you have lots of clutter around your living space, it can still be stressing you out. Experts say that clutter makes us feel weighed down, both literally and figuratively. Too much stuff has been shown to be related to depression, anxiety, self-discipline, and even weight gain. Here's a good rule: If you haven't used something in 12 months, give it away. If shopping is your addiction, consider saving for a retreat of your dreams rather than spending money on material objects. Research shows memorable trips, rather than things, bring us the most happiness.

SLEEP: Are you missing out on those crucial zzz's? Try following the rule of rising with the sun and going to bed when it sets. It may not be so easy to do, but at least aim for a solid eight hours. When sleep deprivation and disturbances become chronic, they increase your risk of developing depression or anxiety disorders. And exhaustion makes it tough to stick to any cleansing program. Aim for an optimum bedtime by curbing your computer, tablet, and smartphone use in the evening.

FEELING COMPETITIVE: Constantly comparing ourselves to others, whether it's our health habits, weight, income, jobs, or possessions, is one of the reasons Americans are not as happy as folks in other countries. What to do if you're just naturally competitive? Focus on being grateful for what you *do* have. Studies show that simple exercises—such as keeping a "gratitude journal" or writing a letter of thanks to a loved one—are associated with greater satisfaction, optimism, and happiness.

THINKING IN A LOOP: Turning the same anxious or fearful thoughts over and over again in your mind sends your body and brain into the stressed-out state known as "fight or flight." It will make your breath and heart rate quicken, and your body release the stress hormones adrenaline and cortisol, all of which takes a toll on both your physical and emotional health. Learn to recognize the thoughts you dwell on most and train yourself to avoid those obsessive pathways. Deep breathing helps. Snapping a rubber band worn on your wrist also works as a reminder to "snap out of it." Meditation helps too because you can practice watching your thoughts arise and then letting them go.

DENYING ANGER: Anger and frustration are both completely normal reactions to life's inevitable challenges. But when you suppress those feelings and let your grudges and grievances fester, it can backfire. Several studies found that suppressed anger is associated with depression. It's important to express negative emotions, but only in appropriate ways. If you can communicate your anger in an assertive but calm manner, you're likely to feel better afterward. If that's not an option, your best bet might be to practice letting it go. Research suggests the act of forgiving offers mental health benefits.

STAYING INDOORS: Not only will staying inside deprive you of crucial vitamin D—it's produced by the body in response to sunlight and has been shown to protect against depression—but being out in nature soothes our souls. Brain scans show that people who walk outside in nature are calmer and less frustrated than when they walk along busy city streets. If you work in an office, take a walk in a green space, if possible, or just sit anywhere outside during your lunch break; it's better than nothing. Just 15 minutes will make a big difference.

OVERWORKING: Speaking of working, a 2011 study of British civil servants found that working 11 or more hours a day (versus a more reasonable 7 or 8), more than doubled a person's odds of sliding into depression. Consider your values and priorities carefully and create a schedule that reflects them. Set aside time for family, friends, hobbies, and healthy habits, like yoga and meditation, with the same seriousness you commit to a meeting at work.

ISOLATION: Although solitude can deepen your spiritual experience and help you to stick to a cleansing diet, withdrawing for any length of time from friends and family is harmful to your well being. By the same token, strong relationships tend to protect against depression and promote happiness. Open your heart and time to those who are important to you.

PERFECTIONISM: Are you trying to meet an unattainably high standard of perfection in everything you do, including maintaining a detox cleanse? Well, that could be a recipe for disappointment and low self-esteem. Perfectionism has been linked to depression, anxiety, and eating disorders. Set real and attainable goals for being healthy. Also, welcome mistakes as avenues for learning, and, most of all, remember to enjoy the journey, not just the destination.

BOOST YOUR POSITIVITY WITH POST-CLEANSE AFFIRMATIONS

- I can't tailor-make the situations in my life but I can tailor-make my attitudes to fit those situations.

- I can change my future by changing my attitude.

- The ultimate measure of who I am is not where I stand in moments of comfort, but where I stand in times of challenge.

- If I don't like something, I can change it by changing the way I think about it.

- Attitudes are contagious. Are mine worth catching?

- My greatest glory is not in succeeding, but in rising up every time I fail.

- You yourself, as much as anybody in the entire universe, deserve your love and affection.

- My strength often increases in proportion to the obstacles imposed upon it.

- No one can make you feel inferior without your consent.

- I am fine just the way I am.

None of these fits just right? Create your own affirmations!

Okay, so who stopped the payment on my reality check?

Be Real: Practice Simple Rules for Digestion

In order to help you stay on a healthy dietary track, here are several simple tips:

CHEW SLOWLY: This is especially necessary when you're eating starches. If you don't, your digestion will become sluggish. You want your starches to get as much saliva as possible so that your gastric enzymes don't have to work on overtime. Some folks like to chew each bite 20 times or more. That's up to you.

AVOID PROCESSED FOODS: It's been said before but is worth repeating. On top of being loaded with chemicals, processed foods are usually packed with sugar: corn syrup, dextrose, sorbitol, lactose (the sugar in milk), etc. You may find it easier to give up junk food after your cleanse. Confession: I found it hardest to forfeit gummy bears. Everybody has their beloved poison. Be easy on yourself if you slip up.

LIMIT PROTEIN: Even the lean kind. Most Americans are too focused on protein and eat more than our bodies need. As a general guideline, the USDA's RDA for protein for adults is 0.8 grams per kilogram of body weight per day. The USDA's average requirement of protein for women ages 31 to 50 is 46 grams per day.

OPT FOR WHOLE GRAINS: The fiber in whole grains helps prevent constipation, a common and aggravating problem. It also helps prevent diverticular disease (the development of tiny pouches inside the colon that are easily irritated and inflamed) by decreasing pressure in the intestines. Overall, most studies show a connection between eating whole grains and better health. Eating whole instead of refined grains substantially lowers total cholesterol, low-density lipoprotein (LDL or bad) cholesterol, triglycerides, and insulin levels.

EAT RAW CHEESE: Who doesn't love cheese? But commercial cheeses may have preservatives and hormones in them. What to do? Eat it raw! According to *U.S. News & World Report*, consumption of raw milk and cheese significantly lowers the symptoms of allergic reactions such as asthma, hay fever, and eczema. Raw milk and its cheese also contain some healthy bacteria which colonize the digestive tract and compete with undesirable pathogens for nutrients. This prevents the growth of the pathogens and reduces the risk of certain infections, according to the Department of Environmental Studies at Macalester College in St. Paul, Minnesota.

Be Real: Consider Food Combining

The philosophy behind food combining is pretty simple. It's based on the fact that our bodies digest foods at different rates and in the process requires different enzymes to break down the foods we eat.

Ten Food Combining Rules

1   PROTEIN AND STARCH: Separate concentrated proteins like meat, fish, and eggs from starches like bread, potatoes, and rice. Why? The body begins by producing the alkaline enzyme ptyalin when a starch is chewed. This begins to break down the starch, but when the food reaches the stomach, the presence of this alkaline enzyme prevents the digestion of proteins in the stomach by pepsin and other acidic stomach

secretions. The result is a heavy, bloated feeling, gas, and toxic wastes bleeding into the blood stream.

2   PROTEIN AND PROTEIN: Avoid meals that combine multiple concentrated proteins, such as fish and cheese, meat and milk, or meat and eggs. Why? Different proteins require different processes to digest. For example, when meat is consumed, the strongest enzymatic reaction occurs during the first hour, whereas milk or eggs take longer to be digested.

3   STARCH AND ACID: Separate starches and acids at mealtime, avoiding combinations like cereal and orange juice, or rice with any vinegar dish. Why? When an acidic food is taken with a starch, the secretion of ptyalin in the mouth is disturbed and the alkaline enzyme needed to break down the starch is absent when the food reaches the stomach.

4   PROTEIN AND ACID: Avoid meals that combine concentrated proteins and acidic dishes. Why? Proteins require acids present in the stomach to digest properly, but adding more acidic foods disrupts the stomach's ability to produce the acid that breaks down protein.

5   PROTEIN AND FAT: Separate concentrated proteins and fatty foods when possible. Why? Fats inhibit the stomach's ability to produce gastric juices, greatly slowing the digestion of any foods taken with the fatty food, especially proteins.

6   PROTEIN AND SUGAR: Combining proteins and sugars together in the same meal should be avoided. Why? Sugar prohibits the stomach's ability to produce gastric juices and so it passes through the stomach to be processed in the small intestine. When combined with a concentrated protein, sugar inhibits the digestion of the protein. This causes fermentation in the gut and an explosion of bacteria, which are both highly toxic to the body.

7   STARCH AND SUGAR: Eat sugars and starches separately. Why? When sugar and starches are combined in the mouth, the

secretion of ptyalin, the alkaline enzyme required for digestion of starches, is halted and starches remain undigested. Sugar fermentation in the gut creates acidic compounds that further inhibit the digestion of starches.

8 MELONS: Consume melons alone or not at all. Why? Melons are a unique food in that they are not digested within the stomach, but pass instead to the small intestine for digestion. This process is only possible when melons are consumed alone or combined only with fresh, raw foods.

9 RAW MILK: Raw milk is to be taken by itself, or not at all. Why? Many people feel that milk should be avoided entirely, but that if consumed it's best in raw form, as pasteurization destroys the natural enzymes in the milk that make its digestion possible.

10 DESSERTS: Sweet, starchy desserts, as well a sweet fruits should not be consumed within a few of hours after large meals containing carbohydrates or concentrated proteins. Why? Sweets after a big meal can interrupt the digestion of almost anything else in the stomach, especially so with carbohydrates and proteins.

Be Real: Stay Beautiful Inside and Out

Posture Points

When it comes to showing our age, posture is a big giveaway. As we get older, it's common for the head and chest to curl inward, the spine to scrunch into the letter "C," and the pelvis to tilt forward. That's not all. A study conducted at the University of Leeds, UK, discovered a connection between muscles in the neck and a part of the brainstem that regulates blood pressure and heart rate. When thrown out of whack it may affect your heart. Also, when your posture is poor your rib cage gets compressed and your internal organs press against your lungs, keeping them from expanding efficiently. The result? Less oxygen in your blood. Conversely, good posture turns all this around. Standing correctly helps your organs work well while you appear more vital, energetic, and confident.

There are a few ways you can help improve your posture:

BALLOON TECHNIQUE: Stand up with your best posture. Now imagine there is a balloon on a string extending from the crown of your head and that this balloon is pulling your head upward toward the sky. Continue doing this for a few weeks and the habit should stick.

GET OUT OF THE CHAIR: It's a fact of life—sitting promotes slouching. As our muscles tire of being in the same position we slump down. Make a habit of getting up and moving, even if just for a minute, once every 30 minutes. Also, get a chair with sufficient lumbar support. This means your chair's backrest should have natural curve that fits into the hollow of your lower back. Basically when sitting down your spine should be in contact with the backrest from your tailbone right up to your upper back.

NIX HIGH HEELS: Heels alter the body's center of gravity and throw it out of alignment. If heels are a must, consider the smaller types.

USE REMINDERS: Visual reminders to stand up tall really work. For example, if you sit at a desk a lot, make a sketch on a Post-it Note of a stick figure standing strait up.

CHECK IT OUT: Use a mirror to align your ears, shoulders, and hips. Proper alignment places your ears loosely above your shoulders and above your hips. Again, although these points make a straight line, the spine itself curves in a slight "S." Look at your side view in a mirror to be sure you're not forcing your back into an unnatural position.

BE TALL IN THE DRIVER'S SEAT: Make sure to sit straight, with your hips pressed against the back of your seat as far as possible. You should be able to hold the steering wheel with your elbows slightly bent.

TELL YOUR BUDS: Ask them to remind you if they catch you slouching.

Ear Coning

Ear coning has long been used in ancient China, Tibet, and other Eastern countries and has recently been gaining popularity in the West. Ear cones, or ear candles, are used to rid your ears of built-up toxins. Many health practitioners, such as colonic therapists, nutritional consultants, and iridologists, have been recommending the use of beeswax ear cones for years. Here's how it works: When the large end of the cone is lit and the small end of the cone is positioned in the ear, the smoke filters into the ear canal, warming the ear wax. As the oxygen in the ear is absorbed by the flame, a gentle vacuum is produced, pulling out the excess wax or foreign material from the ear canal and capturing it in the stem of the ear cone. After the procedure and when the flame is extinguished, the cone can be cut with scissors and the wax or debris can be seen.

Slimming Bath

If you've fallen off conscious eating, there's a chance your body has started to retain water. No worries! This bath concoction will not only smooth and tone your skin but help release the water buildup in your tissues. Simply mix together 20 drops of juniper-lemon or sandalwood-geranium and 20 drops of olive oil. Then put 20 drops of the mixture into a warm bath.

Foot Fix

If your feet are swollen, soak them in a basin of lukewarm water containing six drops of juniper and four drops of lemon oil until the water becomes cool. Use a pumice stone to remove dry skin and soften calluses. Then massage your feet and ankles with upward strokes.

Yoga: Sun Salutation Pose (Surya Namaskar)

In honor of new days and new beginnings, as well as faith in a bright future, the Sun Salutation is ideal.

Stand at the front of your mat in Mountain Pose, with your feet hip-width apart and your weight evenly distributed between them, your spine erect, and your arms at your sides.

Inhale while extending your arms overhead, bringing your palms together, and expanding your chest. For an extra stretch, arch your spine slightly backward into the Crescent Moon Pose—but don't overdo it or you might strain your lower back.

Exhale into the Standing Forward Bend, bringing your chest toward your thighs and your hands toward the floor.

Inhale into Lunge Pose, placing your hands on the mat on either side of your right foot as you lunge your left leg straight back behind you. Expand your chest as you lengthen your spine. Be sure your bent knee is aligned directly above your heel; if it juts out over your toes it might cause too much strain on your knee.

Exhale into Plank Pose, stepping your right leg back so your feet are now side by side. Look straight at the floor, keeping your arms extended and your body straight. Hold this pose for three full breaths.

On an exhale slowly drop your knees to the floor. Untuck your toes, bring your hips back to your heels, and lower your head to the floor with your arms still extended in front of you.

Inhale, slowly bringing yourself up on all fours.

Exhale, slowly bending your elbows and lowering your chest and chin to the floor so your hands, knees, and feet are touching the mat.

Inhale into Upward-Facing Dog Pose, pushing your head and ribcage up off the mat by fully extending your arms as you press the tops of your feet into the ground. Your thighs and hips should rise a few inches above the mat. If you do not have the upper body strength for this pose, lower your knees to the ground, but don't let your hips sag to touch the mat.

Exhale into Downward-Facing Dog Pose, tucking your toes and lifting your hips up and back so that you're bearing your weight on the balls of your feet. This should create an upside-down V shape with your body. Relax your neck and allow the weight of your head to lengthen your spine.

Inhale into the Lunge Pose again, stepping your left foot forward.

Exhale into the Standing Forward Bend again, stepping your right foot forward next to your left foot so your weight is on both feet.

Inhale your arms over your head again.

Exhale, completing the Sun Salutation by returning to Mountain Pose.

Don't forget this *super-important* rule: Drink plenty of purified water!

Grounding Meditation

"It is essential to remember that the aim of meditation is self-awareness, not a state of bliss that is free from problems and obstacles. If we simply seek ecstasy, and hope to avoid sorrow and suffering, then we are actually seeking the loss of ourselves," says Dr. Swami Shankardev Saraswati, a medical doctor and Yoga Master in the Satyananda tradition. "The ultimate aim of meditation is to remain grounded in self-awareness under all conditions of joy and sorrow, pleasure and pain, gain and loss."

Grounding is the process of bringing your awareness into balance along with your body into the present moment.

To achieve this, sit in a comfortable position with a straight spine. Whatever arises in your mind, label it as "just a mental process." Try to keep your awareness as an observer of the process rather than becoming caught up in the mental states themselves. Now take two or three deep breaths, relaxing your body with every exhale. When you're ready, take in a deep breath and visualize your favorite warm, calming color. Feel the color fill every cell of your being, radiating out and around you. Breathe out, letting all the tension go. Breathe in your color again, this time breathing deep down into your belly, your solar plexus. Breathe out, letting all the tension go. Breathe in your color again, this time breathing deep down into the ground, making a solid connection with Mother Earth beneath your seat. Breathe out, letting all the tension go. Keep breathing in and out, feeling the ground beneath you and watching your thoughts come and go.

Are You Keeping It Real?

PART ONE: YOUR BODY

1 You're spending the weekend in a secluded cabin nestled beside a lake in the forest. You pack:
   a. Hiking boots and a swimsuit
   b. A journal
   c. Your cell phone and laptop

2 When the alarm rings in the morning, you:
   a. Lie awake making a mental list of activities for the day
   b. Rise immediately, wondering what the day will bring
   c. Press the snooze button and pull the covers over your head

3   For your birthday you'd rather have:
    a. A surprise party thrown in your honor
    b. Dinner in your favorite restaurant with a loved one
    c. Amnesia

4   At the end of a working day, you feel:
    a. A little beat but ultimately satisfied with your accomplishments
    b. Glad that you can start really living
    c. Exhausted and desperate to relax

5   Which of these statements sounds most like you?
    a. When I'm feeling distressed, I talk it over with a friend or loved one.
    b. Often I feel apprehensive or irritable, and I just don't know why.
    c. I refuse to let myself feel down.

6   Honestly, when you're grocery shopping, does your cart have a
    higher proportion of:
    a. Fruits and veggies
    b. Convenience foods like frozen entrées
    c. Cookies and ice cream

7   Do you drink water:
    a. Whenever you feel thirsty
    b. To meet the recommended quota of eight 8-ounce glasses per day
    c. Not often enough

8   Which of these activities most appeals to you:
    a. Swimming
    b. Sailing
    c. Snoozing

9   Choose the Saturday afternoon closest to your ideal:
    a. Taking a long walk or going to yoga
    b. Time with friends or family
    c. Just hanging out with nothing on your plate

10 Do you stay up late when there's something you want to watch on
    TV even if you're tired:
    a. Rarely
    b. Sometimes
    c. Frequently

11 When you're not on a cleanse, do you mostly crave:
   a. Protein
   b. Complex carbohydrates
   c. Sugar

12 You usually keep your daily schedule:
   a. Partly booked but with some empty spaces
   b. Flexible — to change with your mood
   c. Sacred — you never break plans

13 You feel you're most rested after how many hours of sleep?
   a. 6 hours or fewer
   b. Between 6 and 8
   c. 9 hours or more

PART TWO – YOUR MIND

1 After an argument is resolved, do you find yourself still going over your position in your mind?
   a. Never
   b. Sometimes
   c. Often

2 When you think back on recent conversations, how often do you wish you'd said something else?
   a. Rarely
   b. Sometimes
   c. Often

3 Which method do you most often use when making a decision?
   a. Go with my gut
   b. Weigh the pros and cons
   c. Try to leave the options open

4 How often do you check the news?
   a. Maybe once a day
   b. In the morning and evening
   c. Hourly if possible, but at least several times a day

5   When you buy your best friend a birthday gift, you:
    a. Know in your heart what she would like
    b. Shop around until you find something that's right
    c. Ask her what she really wants

6   When it comes to making plans for the day, you usually:
    a. Go with the flow
    b. Make a list and try to stick to it
    c. Reprioritize and often reconsider plans

Analysis — Your Body

Mostly A's

A spinning top with sparks of energy flying in every direction, you can keep going without taking a break. You join the approximately 20 percent of the American population who fall into the category of Type-A personality, with a naturally speedy metabolism and upbeat attitude that keeps you surging ahead. In order to stay centered, you need to rebalance. Here's how to moderate your energy so you can keep going without burning out:

- ❧ Get enough shut-eye. Although you might need less sleep than most, try to get bed at the same time each night and awake the same time in the morning. Research shows everyone (even you!) needs at least 7 hours of sleep to function efficiently.

- ❧ Take a vitamin B complex supplement. This stress-reducing vitamin keeps your energy humming.

- ❧ Cut out caffeine; you don't need it. Or limit yourself to one cup a day. Try soothing herb teas instead.

Mostly B's

Since moderation is your motto, you try to pace yourself.
To others it might appear that your accomplishments are
effortless, but that's because you can tame your tough
problems by neither getting caught up nor wasting valuable
energy. You keep stuff in perspective. This comes naturally
to you because your metabolism, adrenal glands, and body
type are all set to release energy moderately and without
radical highs or lows. But there are rare occasions when even
you get stressed out and lose your grounding. Recognize
the signs: exhaustion, headaches, backaches, short temper, or
sleeplessness. That's when it's time for you to relax and try
these proven rejuvenation techniques:

- ❧ Acupinch. Apply slight pressure and rub your outer
  ear with your thumb and first finger. This ancient
  acupressure point is a prime meridian for relaxing
  muscle tension from the body.

- ❧ Breathe deeply for 60 seconds and watch your breath.
  This technique sends oxygen to your brain cells,
  giving your mood and thinking power a boost!

- ❧ Take a catnap. Studies show just a 10 minute
  afternoon snooze can be as beneficial as an hour's
  worth of extra sleep.

Mostly C's

Soaking in a warm bath or snoozing on the couch is your
idea of heaven and indeed, it's a healthy practice to set aside
time to relax. But if you allow yourself to spend too much
time in your mind and not enough in your body, it's hard
to get stuff done and meet your goals—which in turn can

trigger the blues. It can become a cycle that takes you out of the joy of the here and now: Low energy leads to sadness and sadness leads to low energy. Other factors? A lag in energy can be caused by a toxic diet, lack of fresh air and light, or too little exercise. Whatever the underlying cause, here are simple grounding techniques:

- Salute the sun three times and get the benefits of mood-boosting light and exercise. You can do these simple yoga stretches in front of a window or outside.

- Take a walk. Studies show just 20 minutes a day outdoors can speed your metabolism and uplift your mood.

- Feel your feelings. When stressful situations arise, be authentic with your feelings: let go of blame and keep your attention on what feels good.

- Put it in writing. According to a University of California study, subjects who kept a daily gratitude journal rated 75 percent higher on scales measuring happiness and reported feeling revitalized and full of energy.

Analysis — Your Mind

Mostly A's

Since you trust the cues you pick up, you move through your days mostly with ease. Life for you means not taking very much seriously. In an existential sense, it's all good. But in reality, sometimes coming to a decision too impulsively or with a lackluster approach can lead to problems down the road. Reduce the possibilities of mistakes by:

- ❧ Sleeping on it. Research shows we can actually problem-solve in our sleep and awake with the best solution.

- ❧ Getting a second opinion. You're used to going it alone, but the old adage "two heads are better than one" is true.

Mostly B's

It's not uncommon for you to question the motives behind the things you and your family and friends say. But this can lead to more questions. To break the cycle:

- ❧ Look for distractions. When you begin overthinking, get up and change places. Studies show that could be enough to switch your thought process.

- ❧ Keep a hand-written "stop" sign on your desk. Visual cues can cut down on excessive thinking.

Mostly C's

A perfectionist and overthinker, it's easy for small issues to avalanche into big problems for you — and then letting go is tough. You can get flooded with worries that swirl around and around, making it difficult for you to resolve problems and stay in the present.

- ❧ Envision a happy ending. Praying or meditating on a positive outcome will block negative thoughts.

- ❧ Steer clear of "worry buddies," friends you know overthink just like you. Reaching out to a positive thinker can help you think positively too.

Final Thought

Partaking in the Yoga-Body Cleanse and renewing your precious self is not a one-time, or even two-time, event. Instead, it's a new way of maneuvering through your world. Once you're aware of toxicity and temptations, and you've gained the tools and commitment to change the way you live, a new and beautiful reality opens. Now you're fully alive.

Be joy!

INDEX

Acknowledgments

Special thanks to Ulysses and my shining star editor, Katherine Furman; Margarita Morello, for her generous spirit and ability to manage whatever is needed; Laurel Marx forever best friend; my son, Gabe, who shows me the way; and to my soul mate, Dr. Bebop, whose patience, musical notes, elegance, courage, and kindness astounds.

About the Author

ROBIN WESTEN received an Emmy Award for the ABC health show *FYI*. She is currently the medical director for Thirdage.com, the largest health site for baby boomers on the Web. She is the author of *Ten Days to Detox*, the *Harvard Medical School Guide Getting Your Child to Eat (Almost) Anything*, as well as *V is for Vagina*, which is coauthored with Alyssa Dweck, MD. She's written feature articles for dozens of national magazines including *Glamour*, *Vegetarian Times*, *Psychology Today*, *SELF*, *Cosmopolitan*, and others. Robin has been practicing yoga, meditation, and cleansing for over fifteen years. She divides her time between Brooklyn and Vermont.